SHATTERED

Published and distributed by Soul Speak Press.
Alexandria, USA

Library of Congress Control Number: 2025908498
Myers, Caitlin
Shattered From Wreckage to Resilience: A memoir of how I reclaimed my life

ISBN
Paperback 978-1-958472-15-6
eBook 978-1-958472-16-3

This work is nonfiction and, as such, reflects the author's memory of her experiences.

SHATTERED

FROM WRECKAGE TO RESILIENCE:
A MEMOIR OF HOW I RECLAIMED MY LIFE

CAITLIN MYERS

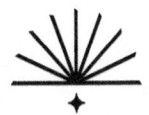

CONTENTS

AUTHOR'S NOTE

This memoir is a tapestry of memories, both my own and those shared with me over the years. Many of these moments are drawn from journal entries I kept throughout my recovery, capturing the raw and intimate details of the journey. The truth is, I was unconscious during much of the initial trauma, and my earliest recollections are fragmented flashes of consciousness—small but vivid pieces that helped me weave this story together.

Much of what I know about those early days comes from conversations with my family, doctors, and nurses, whose perspectives filled in the gaps of what I could not remember. Some parts of my story, however, only came to light as I began the process of writing this book, uncovering details I had never fully understood.

I want to acknowledge that certain parts of this book deal with sensitive subjects, including verbal and physical abuse and other painful experiences. The language in some sections reflects the harsh reality of those moments, though I have intentionally toned down some of the bad language, as this is not the direction I wanted to take with my book. In truth, the sections depicting verbal abuse were even worse than I have portrayed, but I have chosen to soften them while still honoring the truth of my experience.

To my family and friends, my surgeon, the medical team, and those who stood behind the scenes—thank you. I am eternally grateful for your care and support. And to my husband, thank you for letting me write "just one more page."

ONE

GOING BACK

I feel nauseous. I am going to vomit.

My eyes pop open, and I can't see anything clearly with my blurred vision. *Where am I?* I try to roll to my side, my bowels are begging to be released onto the floor, but I can't move because my hands and feet are restrained to the rails on each side of the bed. Realizing I am going to have to vomit on myself, I move to open my mouth and release the nausea onto my chest. Panic takes hold as I quickly realize my mouth is wired together—the confusion I woke up with is only magnified. Morbidly curious about my new circumstance, I go into default mode and instantly run a self-diagnostic on my body. My tongue immediately reaches for the inner parts of my mouth. It retracts in horror when I realize there are tiny wires poking out from both my upper gums and lower. My jaws are being held together by wire, and as I attempt to move my jaws, just a fraction of an inch, panic engulfs me when I realize I cannot open my mouth.

Out of instinct, I try to yell for help, for my mom, for anyone who might be nearby, but I can't move my jaw at all, and only little muffled grunts escape. The left half of my face feels as if I have been at the dentist all morning. Fear begins to take hold as tears stream down my face; I try again to murmur something, make enough noise through my wired jaw, to garner some help. My hands turn into tight little fists as I attempt to break free from the restraints holding me to my hospital bed. Every inch of me is stuck. I can't hold the vomit back any longer. With nowhere to go, the sour taste fills my mouth, seeping through my teeth, backing up through my nose. I try to scream again, but it is as if I am drowning in my own disgusting bile. For as long as I could remember, I carried around an ominous fear of drowning. As my eyes search wildly for help, I understand I now have a front row seat to my personal horror show. I'm going to choke to death on my own vomit. And I don't know why I'm here or how I got here. Hot tears are now streaming in torrents down my face as I continue to make the only sound I can; only a faint, guttural moan, from deep inside my belly is all I can muster, but it is no use—no one will ever hear me. Fight or flight kicks in and my heart is about to push through my already cracked sternum. I cry out to God in my mind as loudly as I possibly can, *Please, someone, anyone, help me!* My body wretches once again and I know the truth of it: This is it, I am going to die. As my eyes begin to slide closed in surrender to my fate, a nurse casually rounds the corner of the door to my room and freezes. To this day, I'm still not sure if it was the shock of seeing me awake for the first time in over a week or the disgusting sight of vomit, spittle, and tears pouring and pooling onto my chest that causes the panic in her eyes to become so clear—even as I lay dying, I can see it. I must give her credit because when she registers what is happening, she moves quickly to the side of my bed reassuringly repeating, "I've got you! I've got you!" She reaches for something over my head, and I hear the rip of masking tape. Her hands return to my line of vision with a pair of pliers that had been taped on the wall directly over my bed. They look like a tool you might use to mend a wire fence on a farm. She quickly begins to clip the wire knots attached to the rods embedded in my upper and lower gums. As the metal is clipped away, I assist by prying my mouth open with the power of my jaw muscles, but something doesn't feel right. As she clips the final wire, my mouth flaps open like a door that hasn't been open in years. The nurse skillfully places her hand behind my head for support as she tips it forward in the only direction it could move. Vomit pours out of me, as if I am a pitcher filled with milk. It goes all over me, soiling my gown and the side of the bed.

"I've got you, it's okay," she whispers as I gasp and wretch and sob. The wires have been holding my jaw to my cranium. The relief of the purge quickly makes room for new pain. The quick and jerking movements compounded onto my broken jaw lead to a pain so intense it radiates across the left side of my face, causing it to feel like it is on fire. As my body tenses for another round of retching, my world goes dark once again. As I fade, I wonder if I am really in hell.

As I lose consciousness, the nurse works swiftly. I will never forget her touch, so gentle; she treated my broken body with the same tender care she would deliver to a newborn baby. It would be many weeks later, but I would learn a nurse was assigned to my side—and meant to be there every minute of every day—due to my critical situation and the high risk of aspirating. She not only treated me with a humbling amount of dignity that day, but she saved my life.

EARLY CHILDHOOD

I was raised in quintessential small-town USA, tucked away in Northwest Florida—where the locals say it's more "lower Alabama" than the Sunshine State. Life moves slowly, wrapped in the embrace of Southern hospitality, where neighbors wave from their front porches and everyone knows your business before you do. I was found frequenting the beach with friends and family often, soaking in the emerald-green waters and digging my toes into the sugar-white sand. It was a forty-five-minute drive from my house, just far enough to make the trips feel like an adventure but close enough that it always felt like a part of home.

Even as a child, I was a fiercely vocal, type A personality. My cousin and I proudly declared ourselves the leaders of the "RA Club," or Radical Attitude Club, where the only requirement for membership was wearing a Calvin Klein hat and attending our meetings in the upstairs bonus room of my grandparents' house.

I was headstrong and stubborn, traits often associated with middle-child syndrome, and frequently seen stomping around in my worn-out turquoise cowgirl boots paired with a vintage gold sequin vest—an outfit as bold as my personality. In old photos and snippets of home videos, I see a bundle of sass and boundless curiosity. But there was another side to me too. I had a soft spot for the broken, the fragile. Stray animals, injured birds, the lizard that got its tail caught in my great-grandmother's door—I was their first responder, tucking tiny creatures into my pockets, determined to rehabilitate them with whatever scraps of care I could manage. And when they didn't make it, I staged elaborate funerals under the large oak tree that held our tire swing on my grandfather's property next to our house. The ceremonies were complete with eulogies and gravestones made of rocks, dragging my sister along as an unwilling mourner.

Like many young girls, I went through a tomboy phase. I was interested in everything from building forts in the woods to coed soccer to shooting rifles with my dad and grandfather. At just twelve years old, I proudly shot my first deer, though I couldn't help but cry afterward. Growing up in a family of avid hunters, it felt like a rite of passage—a moment that was both bittersweet and deeply rooted in our family traditions.

I was fiercely protective of my friends and family and did not tolerate bullying of any kind. My cousin Blakely likes to jokingly remind me of when we were in second grade playing on the playground at the Christian school we attended. She suddenly screamed as a young boy tried to hold her down. At full speed, I sprinted in her direction and sucker punched the poor boy square in the face. That was the first and only time I was ever sent to the principal's office. I was small but mighty and wore my heart on my sleeve. My parents like to tease that every gray hair on their head came from me. I guess there is some truth to that. My dad would say, "Oh, I got some new gray hair today! Thanks, Caitlin!"

My dad coached several sports, one being track, and often tried to recruit me when he witnessed my lightning speed as I raced my brother in our backyard. My siblings and I had a toughness instilled in us at a young age and we were all very competitive. I was always very proud of the fact that I could beat most of the boys in our school relay races. One day I was given the nickname "Legs" due to my speed and large calf muscles, a nickname that grew on me over the years.

When I entered ninth grade, my schedule quickly filled with extracurricular activities, including joining the weightlifting team. Strength training became my passion—I loved the challenge of pushing my body to its limits. The weightlifting coach noticed my potential early on, impressed by the amount I could lift despite my small frame. I'll never forget my first meet, going head-to-head against a team who completely outmatched us. I can still remember the sharp focus it took, the weight of the bar in my hands, and the muffled sound of my teammates shouting "Legs!" somewhere in the background.

In what felt like the blink of an eye, my senior year arrived, bringing with it the daunting question of what came next. Like most of my friends, I chose to stay local for college and enrolled at the University of West Florida (UWF). Uncertain of my career path, I drifted for awhile, trying to figure out who I was and who I wanted to become. With a family full of educators, it seemed natural to follow in their footsteps. I applied for a substitute teaching position with the Florida Department of Education, completed the certification process, and began filling in for grades ranging from kindergarten to twelfth grade.

At first, I loved the idea of making a difference—helping a child learn something new or inspiring them in some small way. But as the weeks went by, it became clear that teaching wasn't where my heart was. While I stuck with it for the rest of the year to earn some extra cash, I couldn't ignore the pull toward something else. I wanted a career where I could help people in a way that felt more aligned with my passions. Naturally, I gravitated toward health and wellness, a perfect fit given my love of fitness and self-care.

In my last year of college, I was breezing through my elective classes, my favorite was taken alongside my best friend Dawna. Somehow, she had convinced me to take a soldering class with her, even though I did not know the first thing about fusing pieces of hot, liquid metal together. We soon found ourselves seated side-by-side, in the small workshop-like studio that sat adjacent to the main art building. Classroom hours quickly turned into social hour for us. We spent most of our time chatting about our hopes and aspirations after college. Plans to travel kept popping up in conversation, which caused us to organize a post-graduation trip to Arizona. We shared a love for the outdoors, so this was perfect. Soldering was quickly placed on the backburner as researching our trip to Arizona became the focus. The possibility of immersing ourselves in the awe-inspiring landscapes, enjoying the authentic local cuisine, and hiking the Grand Canyon from rim-to-rim caused these two, small-town college girls to wish the rest of their college days away.

During this time, my body felt unstoppable, like it had been carved out of pure momentum. Fitness wasn't just something I did—it was the thing I craved, the thing I fed on. My drug of choice wasn't alcohol or late-night parties; it was the flood of dopamine, endorphins, and adrenaline that surged through me after a grueling workout. I kept up my weightlifting routine throughout college, joined the UWF running club to add some variety, and even picked up a part-time job at a local fitness center. Somehow, that led to filming commercials for Max Muscle Nutrition—small-town fame, the kind that felt bigger than it was.

By then, my academic workload had thinned. I'd chipped away at my core classes and found myself with a little more room to breathe, so I doubled down on my passions. I worked toward an advanced fitness certification and reignited a long-dormant dream: dance. All throughout my childhood, I'd dabbled in ballet, jazz, and hip-hop. The thought of joining a professional dance team in Tampa the following spring tugged at something deep in me, a desire to move, to create, to escape the small-town bubble that felt like it might swallow me whole.

The road back to dance wasn't easy. I spent a year squeezing in night classes with a former University of Florida dance instructor into my already packed schedule. She would sigh dramatically at me, half joking but not really, "Caitlin, you're like a freight train coming full speed ahead. I need graceful, fluid motions!" Strength and technique came naturally, elegance, not so much. But I kept at it, laser focused on the goal. The promise of traveling the world with the team—on someone else's dime, no less—lit a fire in me. It wasn't just about dance. It was about adventure. About proving to myself that there was more to life than the limits of what I'd always known.

TWO

SPOTS

My twenty-first birthday is on the horizon, and as always, my friends and I find an excuse to celebrate. Orange Beach, Alabama, becomes the destination of choice. We pack our essentials with the giddy efficiency of college students and pile into my red Mitsubishi Eclipse convertible, the car my dad surprised me with my senior year of high school. Even now, years later, the memory still stirs tears. It wasn't new—it had its share of dings and scrapes—but nothing a little touch up paint couldn't fix. When he handed me the keys, I cried as I threw my arms around his neck, telling him it was perfect. And it was.

We hit the highway, blasting the CD player with our carefully curated playlist—hours spent downloading and burning tracks for this very moment. Lil Wayne and Kenny Chesney bump through the speakers as the wind whips through our hair, and we laugh until our stomachs ache. The kind of laugh that's free and full and makes you feel like nothing could ever go wrong. As we cruise down the highway, I marvel out loud at the small milestone of being old enough to book a hotel room on my own. But age doesn't stretch our budget any further. The Comfort Inn by the beach is the best our thin, college-student wallets can manage.

The room is forgettable—stiff queen-sized beds, a dated floral comforter and a view of the overcrowded parking lot. We toss our bags onto the beds and race to the shore. The day is seventy-five degrees and flawless. The green flag flutters above calm seas, and the salty breeze feels like the perfect welcome. We float and splash, dive and soak, until our bodies are spent and the sun begins to dip below the horizon. Wrapped in oversized towels, we collapse onto the sand and watch as the sky performs its final act. Purple violets bleed into fiery streaks of orange, a kaleidoscope of colors colliding with the gulf. We can't look away. The grandeur is too much, too beautiful.

Since it's my birthday celebration, I decide to trade my usual activewear for something bold—a vibrant green dress, dangling earrings, and my favorite wedge sandals. When I catch a glimpse of myself in the mirror, I can't help but smile. For once, everything about my outfit feels just right. I notice my friend watching me from across the room, a grin spreading across her face. She laughs and gives me a quick thumbs up, her silent seal of approval.

"Taxi's here!" I call out, and the room bursts into chaos. We're like middle schoolers headed to a sleepover, skipping around, grabbing our purses, double-checking our reflections, and laughing until our sides hurt. We pile into the back of the taxi, shoulder to shoulder, buzzing with anticipation. We decide on my favorite Thai restaurant, perched right on the edge of the ocean. The aroma of chicken pad thai greets us as we step inside, warm and familiar.

After dinner, the Florida humidity takes hold, and my hair starts its usual frizz-fight as we make our way to the taxi. Our next stop is a dive bar just down the road, its neon lights flickering like a signal calling us in.

The bar is packed, the band deep into an '80s playlist, and the dance floor is a wild, pulsing mess. We post up in a corner taking it all in. My gaze sweeps over the room until it lands on him. He's tall, confident, and undeniably handsome. He's looking right at me. My stomach flips, and I quickly look away, my heart pounding. When I glance back, his eyes haven't moved. I feel heat rise in my cheeks as I force myself to focus on anything but him.

Before I have time to think, he's moving toward me, weaving through the crowd with an ease that feels practiced. Suddenly, he's there, standing right in front of me. "Want to dance?" he asks, his voice smooth and easy, like he's already sure of my answer. But I freeze. My no-dancing-with-strangers rule screams in my mind, and after a brief hesitation, I shake my head and politely decline.

His eyebrows lift slightly in surprise, but he takes it in stride, giving me a small, understanding smile before walking away. I watch him go, already questioning my decision. I steal glances at him over the next hour, and every time I do, I catch him looking back. My heart races as I pretend not to notice, though I know my face is giving me away.

Then, just as I've convinced myself I imagined it all, he's back. This time, he doesn't waste time with pleasantries. He stands directly in front of me, extends his hand, and says, "Let's try this again. I'm Dave." I pause for only a second before taking his hand. A Division I college football player, he's in town with some of his teammates for spring break. As I listen intently to his introduction, I can't help but think that he is completely my type. I am interested. We chat for a bit longer but then my friends begin to pull me away. "Can I have your cell number?" He quickly asks as my girlfriend continues tugging on my arm. "I'm leaving tomorrow, but I'd like to call you!" I shake myself free from my friend and rattle off my number before he disappears somewhere into the back of the bar.

To my surprise, he calls me the very next day. I tell him I'm not looking for a relationship, but Dave doesn't seem to care. He's persistent, relentless even. Night after night, we talk, his charm seeping through the phone in a way that feels both unexpected and disarming. Before I know it, the lines between just talking and something more blur, and I feel myself falling into the story I swore I wouldn't write.

*   *   *

I check my lipstick nervously in the rearview mirror of my car. After about a year of casual phone calls, Dave finally invites me to dinner with him and a friend. I smooth out my dress as I step out of the car, rehearsing a casual smile. When I walk through the door, our eyes meet, and I immediately take in the scene—two other guys at the table with him. "Hi! How are you?" I ask, sliding into the seat next to him, trying to seem composed. He turns to me with a grin, one that looks playful at first. "That's how you're going to greet me? Like I'm just some guy?" he says, his voice light but laced with something I can't quite place. At the moment, I admire his boldness. He knows what he wants, and it feels refreshing. *Confident*, I think. *Direct*. I'm not sorry that what he seems to want, at least for now, is me.

But as I sit there, something about the moment lingers uncomfortably. Later, when I know him better, I realize it isn't confidence at all. It's embarrassment. Anger, even. He's annoyed that I didn't fawn over him, didn't greet him with a hug or a kiss or whatever grand display he had built up in his head. I've failed to play the role he's written for me, and I can see it now—this is how it starts.

Dave and I keep talking and seeing each other over the next few weeks. It feels like young summer love, the kind you read about, set against the backdrop of Orange Beach. He takes me to all the nicest restaurants and buys the most expensive wine on the menu. Now that he's graduated, Dave lives in his parents' condo overlooking the water—a lavish life compared to my small-town Southern roots.

That summer, things shift. We take our friendship to the next level and start dating exclusively. At first, I tell myself I don't really know what I'm getting into, but maybe that's just an excuse. Dave has a mean streak, one he hides well under a pretense of caring, but it's there, just under the surface. My friends and family see it too. They try to warn me.

"He's off the rails, Caitlin, and I can't stand him. You deserve way better," Dawna says one night over sushi. She's never one to sugarcoat her thoughts, and it's part of why we're close.

"I don't know what to do," I admit, my voice low. "He keeps pulling me back in. I do plan to end it, eventually."

"When?" she asks, her voice rising with urgency. "Tomorrow? He scares me."

"I don't know yet. I'm still figuring out the logistics," I answer softly, looking down at my plate. Dave's name doesn't come up again that evening, but it lingers in the space between us, unspoken but heavy.

A few months into dating, despite objections from almost everyone in my life, Dave invites me to meet his parents. His dad Richard is an accomplished lawyer who runs his own firm. He's tall and broad, the kind of man who commands a room. His light brown hair is thinning, but his face holds a permanent smile that makes me feel welcome. His mom is the quintessential Southern belle, all charm and warmth, her accent wrapping around every "Hey y'all!" she sings out. She's a talented designer and moves through the room with a familiarity that makes her approachable.

That summer, my life feels like a blur. Between working full-time at a dental office and taking summer classes, I barely have time to breathe. Still, I manage to squeeze in a few trips to Orange Beach on the weekends to visit Dave. One of the things I love most about him—at least at first—is that we both share a passion for cooking. We spend hours in his parents' condo cooking up delicious gourmet meals.

One evening, while Dave is out for a run, I decide to surprise him by making dinner on my own. I rush around the kitchen, my heart racing as I scramble to gather ingredients. His runs typically last an hour, and I want everything to be perfect. In my hurry, I accidentally knock over an expensive-looking candle. I freeze for a moment, staring at the shattered glass. Nothing in this house is cheap. I try to salvage it, but the oil in the pan starts to sizzle. I tell myself, it's just a candle—it can wait.

"Is that chicken I smell?" Dave asks as he walks in, sweat dripping from his run.

"Yes, it is!" I reply, trying to sound cheerful. He disappears to shower, and I keep cooking. By the time he comes back, he's settled at the bar, chatting with me while I plate the food. But then his gaze shifts. He sees the broken candle on the counter.

Before I can explain, his voice erupts, sharp and accusing. "What the hell happened to that candle?"

Startled, I try to explain. "I was rushing to make dinner before you got back and knocked it over by accident. I was going to tell you about it."

"No, you weren't," he snaps, cutting me off. "You were clearly trying to hide it!" His voice rises, his words barreling over mine as I try to apologize.

"It was an accident, Dave!" I almost plead.

But he doesn't let up. His sarcasm cuts deeper than his yelling. "Oh, sure. We'll just go buy a new one because we've got all this money, right? Well, guess what? You're going to buy a new candle."

I stare at him, spatula still in my hand. "I wasn't trying to hide that I broke it—I'll always admit to something I've done," I say evenly, meeting his eyes. "It's just a candle. Calm down. And yes, I'll buy a new one."

The smell of burning chicken fills the air as he continues to berate me. Tears sting my eyes, a mix of frustration and fear. All I wanted was to make a nice dinner, but now the evening is ruined. When we finally sit down to eat, the tension is unbearable. Every word feels heavy, every movement cautious, like I'm walking on eggshells, waiting for the next explosion.

Dave never apologizes. I barely touch the charred chicken on my plate, my gaze fixed instead on the sun sinking into the gulf. It's breathtaking, its beauty a stark contrast to the suffocating atmosphere inside this house.

*   *   *

"You're going to wear that?" Dave asks, his tone flat but laced with something sharper. We're in his parents' timeshare in Orlando, and up until this moment, the trip has been smooth, almost enjoyable. The plan for the day is simple: Walt Disney World, starting with Disney's Animal Kingdom Theme Park. I've dressed for comfort—a slicked-back ponytail, minimal makeup, and my trusty black Converse sneakers, the ones that have seen better days but feel like home.

"Yes, I am," I say, my teeth clenched, my voice firm. He wants someone to showcase, someone who glows in curated outfits and delicate heels, and sometimes, I play along. I don't mind dressing up—I enjoy it, even—but only on my terms. Not today. Today, I just want to feel like myself. The thought of conforming to someone else's standards, of being told who to be, feels unbearable.

Dave is a perfectionist, and I've always had a love-hate relationship with that. At first, it felt like ambition, like drive, but now I see it for what it is—control. He nitpicks every little thing: the way I laugh too loud, talk too much, reach for that extra roll at dinner. Every comment chips away at me, makes me feel smaller, like a child being scolded.

I think about the time I left a towel on the bathroom floor after a shower. He called me in and stood there, pointing like I was the family dog that had knocked over the trash. "What's wrong in here?" he asked, his voice mocking. "Excuse me?" I said, staring at him in disbelief. He pointed at the towel, his face twisted in disapproval. "That towel isn't going to pick itself up," he said, his tone thick with condescension. I felt like I'd walked onto the set of *Sleeping with the Enemy.*

When I strip away the excuses, the rationalizations, I know it isn't perfectionism I hate—it's him. Dave is a bully.

After the outfit incident, I'm carrying my mug of coffee through the living room, careful not to spill. Dave is on the couch, glued to his phone, his leg stretched out across the cushions. I realize I've forgotten my phone on the kitchen counter and pivot to grab it. As I turn, Dave extends his foot deliberately, catching mine. I stumble forward, the coffee spilling all over me. He laughs as I hit the floor, his laughter sharp and cruel.

I push myself up, fuming. "Why would you do that?" I snap, brushing myself off. "You're such a jerk, Dave!" He keeps laughing, like my anger is a joke, like I'm a joke.

This is who he is—a man who trips me for fun, who mocks my pain, who makes me feel like I'm too much and not enough all at once.

At dinner that night, he comments on a woman at the bar. She's laughing with her friends, her confidence radiant, her low-cut dress showcasing her perfectly augmented breasts. "When will you get a pair like that?" he says casually, like he's asking me to pass the salt.

I stare at him, stunned. "Not in this lifetime," I say, my voice sharper than I expect.

The days stretch on, and with each one, I feel more tired, more burdened, more like a shadow of myself. My happy-go-lucky spirit, the part of me that once lit up rooms, is gone. I left it back at the rooftop bar where Dave made that comment, or maybe before that. I've lost track.

On the drive home, the car is quiet. I stare out the window, watching the world blur past, and wonder, *Is this it? Is this what I've let my life become?* Dave fills the silence with a one-sided conversation, his words circling, dominating the space, but I barely hear him.

As I sit there, trapped in the quiet violence of my own thoughts, I realize the truth: Every day I stay, this relationship chips away at me. I feel the cracks spreading, the pieces of myself breaking off, becoming lost. I carry with me a maze of doubts, insecurities etched into my skin by his words, his actions.

I don't know how it ends, but I know this much—I can't keep losing myself to him.

*   *   *

That fall I returned to UWF entering my senior year of college. While most couples have arguments and disagreements, ours became more frequent and took on a ferocity that was primal. He became even more controlling and domineering, demanding I account for my every move. In just a few months I went from the excited-about-life college girl to a paranoid shell of myself who was always second guessing my every decision. He tore me to shreds. And it seemed like he enjoyed it.

Despite my trepidation with his behavior, my weekend visits to Orange Beach to see him continued. Over the summer Richard, Dave's father, had traveled down to Florida to talk with Dave and told him that he needed to get a job now that he had graduated college. I think it was his nice way of saying, "Get a job or you will get cut off!" Dave made the decision to attend culinary school in Austin, Texas. It was settled. In two short weeks, he was scheduled to move into a luxury apartment just minutes from downtown Austin. I remember feeling sad he was leaving, but in some ways, it was a relief to see him go. I thought the distance between us might make for an easier breakup.

The weeks flew by. I finally finished midsemester finals and was relieved to be on fall break. Dave was in Texas knee-deep in culinary school with very little free time. I toyed with the idea of driving to see him, but ultimately decided to stay local and enjoy fall break with friends and family. Dave was not thrilled by my wanting to spend my off time away from him. "Why wouldn't you want to come here?" he blurted out through the phone. There was tension in his voice. Continuing in conversation, I was forced to turn the volume down. At one point I just held the phone away from my ear while annoyingly rolling my eyes. "I just don't feel like driving all that way," I said. "Fine! I've got stuff to do and you're just pissing me off!" he said. And with that, he hung up the phone. I had become accustomed to his tantrums and regular berating to the point I began to tune him out.

That night, I texted Dave I was going out with friends and silenced my cell phone. I joined my friends at a cozy restaurant in town. It was a local favorite. I knew Dave was blowing up my phone by now. I didn't care. My aunt, uncle, and brother joined our group later that evening. It was a great time as usual. My family was close knit, and I was thrilled whenever we had an opportunity to spend time together.

The restaurant roared with patrons as we struggled to make conversation, being forced to lean into each other, practically yelling. Even if I hadn't silenced my phone, I wouldn't have heard it. My aunt excused herself from the restroom to make a call. As she pulled out her phone, she realized she had over twenty missed phone calls and several voice messages. In his hysteria at not being able to get a hold of me, Dave had somehow gotten his hands on my aunt's cell number because he knew she was with me. One by one she listened to the list of voicemails in the bathroom, growing increasingly annoyed and concerned. As she reentered the bar, I could tell by her expression that something wasn't quite right, and my heart skipped a beat. She came over to me, and pulled me aside so as not to announce her news to the entire table. "Your boyfriend called me and is very angry. He's looking for you," she said. My face grew hot as she recounted his messages. I couldn't believe it. *The nerve of him. It was one thing to be threatening me, but my aunt?* "Why do you put up with this? You don't deserve to be treated this way," she said.

Flustered, I couldn't seem to muster up a response to my aunt. Instead, I hopped out of my seat and darted to the bathroom. Locked in a stall, I took a deep breath as I reached for my phone. I had over sixty missed calls.

"He is crazy," I mumble to the toilet, the phone barely rings. "Where the hell are you?" he demands. "How dare you not answer your phone? I know you're out whoring around!" Stunned, I sink to the edge of the toilet seat as the accusations continue. *Whoring around? Is that what he considered me doing when I was just enjoying the company of friends and family?* The screaming goes on splashed with regular intervals of expletives, he interrogates me for a solid minute. I don't say a word. Helpless to defend myself, I just let the words fly like daggers, realizing I feel nothing for him. When he has finally lost his voice, I see my opportunity and say only two words: "I'm done!"

"You don't tell me when we are done!" he shrieks with half his voice gone. Like I am building a wall of words to protect me, or perhaps it's a mantra that I need to stay focused on so I can escape this verbal lashing with my resolve in tack, I just keep repeating, "I'm done. I'm done. I'm done!" I slam the phone shut, stand up, smooth my dress with my hands and walk out of the bathroom stall with my head held high. I don't even shed a tear. "I broke it off with him." It was a declaration to the table—one that he must have been imagining because as soon as the words left my mouth, I feel the vibration of my cell phone in my back pocket. I reach for my phone and turn it off for the remainder of the night.

Dave calls relentlessly over the next few weeks. I don't answer. He sends flowers, chocolate covered strawberries, handwritten letters. The text messages grow longer and more desperate, but I delete them all. The flowers go straight into the trash. The letters too. The strawberries? I eat them. Who am I to let dessert go to waste?

I'm working full-time as a dental assistant while finishing college. Most of my classes are online, except for Fridays. My days start before dawn—up at 5:00 a.m., at work by 5:40. Dave knows my schedule like the back of his hand.

It's a Monday, and we're drowning in patients. By the time the last one leaves, I'm exhausted. I'm scrubbing my hands in the sterilization room, lost in my thoughts, when someone taps me on the shoulder. I jump, spinning around with soapy hands, and there he is. Dave. Smiling awkwardly, holding a dozen red roses.

"What are you doing here?" I ask, my voice flat.

"I drove all the way from Texas to see you," he says. His tone is soft, apologetic. I want to be annoyed, but something in me—some old, familiar part of me—feels strangely happy to see him. Against my better judgment, I agree to meet him after work. I tell myself we'll talk things through. Maybe find some resolution now that he's had time to cool off.

That evening, we meet at a local, quiet restaurant. It's a weekday, so we practically have the place to ourselves. Dave speaks with a tone I almost don't recognize, full of regret, full of promises. He apologizes for everything—the fights, the yelling, the way he's treated me. "I know I'm the issue," he says. "I need to change. I can't do it alone though. I don't want to do it without you." His words are everything I want to hear. They plant a tiny, dangerous seed of hope. Maybe this time will be different. Maybe he's finally ready to change. Before I know it, his apology wins me over, and just like that, we're back together.

*   *   *

Dave buys us tickets to a New Year's Eve party in Austin, Texas. I'm excited, almost giddy as we head into the city. I spend the day texting my family and friends, sending pictures of the festivities. Dave isn't happy about it. Every other question is an accusation. "Who are you texting?" "What are you doing on your phone?"

At dinner, he drinks more than usual. He's always been a drinker, but tonight he takes it further. It loosens him up, makes him funnier, more relaxed—until it doesn't. Until he's glaring at a guy across the room for looking at me too long, muttering about how he'll "deal with him" if it happens again.

When the clock strikes midnight, the room erupts in cheers. Champagne glasses clink, and for a moment, everything feels light, hopeful. Dave seems fine. He eats between drinks, keeps it together. But when we get back to the hotel, it unravels. I sit on the edge of the bed, texting my mom a picture of the festive New Year's Eve decor. Dave walks out of the bathroom, zipping his pants.

"What the hell are you doing?" he shouts. His face is red, his voice loud enough to make me flinch.

I stand up, my phone in hand. "I'm texting my mom. Calm down."

"You've been on your phone all night texting some guy, haven't you?" His words are venomous, cutting. Before I can respond, he lunges, knocking the phone out of my hands. I yell, "Have you lost your mind?!" but it only fuels his anger. He takes another step, his accusations flying faster and louder. "You're cheating on me, aren't you? Who is he?"

I don't even have time to defend myself before he's on me. One hand grabs the back of my neck, the other clamps around my throat. He slams me onto the mattress, and I slide off the edge, hitting the floor hard. My head smacks against the wall, and for a moment, the world tilts.

I lay there, stunned, every part of me frozen in fear. Dave towers over me, breathing hard. His eyes meet mine, and for a second, he looks as shocked as I feel. But then he steps closer, and I scramble backward, reaching for my phone. "I'm calling the police!" I scream.

He grabs the phone before I can dial, and then blocks the exit door. I'm defenseless. My heart pounds as I dart for the bathroom, slamming the door and locking it behind me. My hands shake as I sink to the floor, pressing my back against the door. I stay there for what feels like hours, listening to the silence on the other side. I don't dare open the door. Instead, I spread a few towels on the cold tile and curl up, pulling a damp one over me like a blanket. As I drift off, one thought keeps repeating in my head: This is how I'm starting the new year.

When I wake up, stiff and cold, I crack the door open just enough to peek out. Dave is asleep on the bed, fully clothed. I tiptoe around the room, grabbing my things as quietly as I can. My mind races. *I just need to get to my car. If I can make it to my car, I'll be safe.*

Dave stirs as I'm zipping my bag. He looks at me, confused. "What's going on?" he asks.

"We got into a fight," I say, keeping my voice steady. "I slept on the bathroom floor." I make it sound like it's nothing, like this is normal. He frowns, says he blacked out and doesn't remember a thing. I don't push. I just nod and keep packing, my focus on getting out of the hotel room.

We go to breakfast with one of his friends, and for the first time since last night, I feel a small sense of safety being in a public setting. Over coffee, I look him in the eye and say quietly, "You put your hands on me." He denies it, of course. "There's no way I'd do that," he says. Then, in classic Dave fashion, he flips it. "How do I know you didn't put your hands on me?"

It's always the same with him. Deny, deny, counter accuse. In true narcissist fashion, he is never wrong, and there is never any changing his mind.

I make it home in one piece and call off the relationship, again. We go days without talking, but finally Dave breaks the silence when he reaches out, curious about how I am doing. I keep my messages short, direct, and infrequent. Always an avid animal lover, Dave knows what he is doing when he reaches out one day to tell me he has found an injured kitten alongside the road. He asks me for advice on how to care for it, and my frozen heart begins to thaw with every picture he texts of the cutest kitten I've ever seen. After the third picture comes through, he calls. I pick up the phone and we speak at length. "How are you? What have you been up to?" turns into me agreeing to join him for an all-expenses-paid ski trip to Colorado. Visions of slicing through powdery snow in a chic-yet-sporty ski outfit while surrounded by stunning winter scenery suddenly renders me with amnesia regarding New Year's Eve. The bait had been thrown—he knew what I liked and dangled it in front of me.

*　*　*

And just like that, we're off and running again.

I'm tucked into the corner of a leather sofa at the ski lodge in Colorado, marveling at how cozy I feel. Snow piles high outside the window, and I laugh to myself as I watch tiny skiers "pizza" down the bunny slopes, their little bodies wobbling as they try to stay upright. I'm living the dream—a Florida girl in a real winter wonderland. Back home, we only ever got a light dusting of snow, maybe once or twice my entire childhood. This feels like magic.

But the coziness doesn't last. The hot chocolate I'm holding starts to warm me too much, and I can feel sweat pooling under the layers of my oversized red and black ski onesie. I start unzipping it, the heat building with every second, when Dave bursts through the lodge doors.

The smile I have ready for him freezes on my face. His stormy expression hits me first, then the heavy way he slams himself into the chair next to me. His parents trail in behind him, Susan looking like she's stepped straight out of Ski Glamour Weekly—every hair in place, her lipstick perfectly red, her jacket cinched at the waist just so. They don't speak. None of them do. They sit silently in the rustic, mid-century chairs across from me, their presence pressing down on the room like a weighted blanket.

Clearly something's wrong. The warmth I felt just minutes ago is replaced with a cold unease that creeps up my spine. Dave's eyebrows are bunched together, his jaw clenched so tight I can see the muscle twitch. My fingers tap nervously on the wooden coffee table as I wonder what I've done to provoke this. It's always something, isn't it?

Finally, I work up the courage to ask, "Are you okay?"

I barely get the words out before he slams his fist onto the table. The sound reverberates through the lodge as he shouts, "No!" Heads turn. Other patrons pause mid-conversation, craning their necks to see where the outburst came from. Dave shoots up from his chair and storms off, his boots thudding heavily on the wooden floor.

I glance at Susan. Her eyes meet mine, and they're full of something I don't quite know how to name—pity, maybe, or sadness. Richard doesn't even look up. His head stays bowed, his hand rubbing over his forehead like he's trying to erase whatever just happened.

The silence is unbearable. Sweat drips down my back, and I know it's not just the onesie anymore. I have to say something—anything—but the words won't come. Minutes stretch on like hours. Finally, Richard shifts in his chair, turning to look out the window. His shoulders slump, and when he speaks, his voice is low and measured.

"Caitlin," he says, leaning forward, resting his large hands on the table. He waits until I meet his eyes. "A leopard cannot change its spots."

The words hang in the air between us. He doesn't explain. He doesn't need to. We both know exactly who he means. The glint in his eyes, the weight of his tone—it's a warning.

I don't respond. I can't. I drop my gaze back to the coffee table, my mind spinning. When I finally look up again, I force myself to focus on the bunny slopes outside the window. The children are still out there, still learning to pizza, still falling and getting back up.

That night, I lie in bed replaying the scene over and over, trying to make sense of it. My heart aches for Richard and Susan. They don't deserve this any more than I do. Later, Dave admits without much prompting that his tantrum was because he didn't get a Christmas gift from his parents. The ski trip was supposed to be his gift, but it wasn't enough for him. It's never enough for him.

I roll onto my side, clutching my pillow as frustration wells up inside me. Why can't he just be grateful? Deep down, I know the truth. He's not good for me. He never has been. And no matter how much I hope for change, I can't escape Richard's words: A leopard cannot change its spots.

I need to start planning my way out. Fast.

THREE

LAST NIGHT'S MAKEUP

JANUARY 21, 2010

I groggily reach for my phone and tap the screen to check the morning weather forecast for Austin. A groan escapes involuntarily as I register the prediction—a cold day looming and dreary; it matches how I feel when I think about seeing Dave. I make my way to the bathroom, glimpsing at my reflection as I pass the mirror. I stop to take it all in. For the fourth time, I prepare myself to confront him; the playboy boyfriend whose charms and gifts once ensnared my heart but whose cruelty has shattered my spirit. My flight to Austin is on time and scheduled to depart at dusk, and I know, once I hop on that plane, there is no turning back on my decision to go and be with him, despite my reservations.

"It's only three days," I whisper to myself.

As the fading sunlight casts shadows through my window, I quickly select my attire—a black V-neck shirt with a cinched waist, paired with my go-to black boots from Target that fit perfectly snug over a dark pair of blue jeans. My lipstick is a quiet shade of nude, standing as a testament to the silence on my lips—a lack of defiance against the chains binding me to a relationship steeped in toxicity. As I put one more coat of lipstick on, I find it challenging to identify the emotions swirling within me. I am desperate to find the strength to end the cycle of pain once and for all.

I know I shouldn't go, yet here I am, packing my suitcase in preparation for the journey. I add the final clothing items to my suitcase and take note of the butterflies in my stomach; they are so different from the ones I felt when we first started our relationship. No, what I feel now is not exhilarated anxiety. It's a constant pit embedded deep inside my gut, creating fear and dread. My sister leans against the wall with her arms crossed, silently watching me pack my belongings. She doesn't say a word. I notice a look of concern on her face as I reach for my luggage.

"Don't go! I have a bad feeling about all of this," she pleads quietly. I stop, my hand on the handle of my roller bag.

"It's just a quick trip. Plus, I'm planning to break things off with him when I get back," I snap, my voice betraying traces of frustration. Conflicting emotions stir within me, yet I reassure her—and myself—that everything will be fine.

Hurriedly, I wheel my red carry-on suitcase out to my car and make a dash for the airport. Alarm bells keep going off in my head. I have a premonition that something bad will happen if I go. I am scared. I feel like I have no choice—Dave surprised me with the plane ticket for his birthday weekend, and I don't want to upset him by refusing his offer. In this moment, I realize I have become so consumed with making Dave happy that I have lost touch with my own desires and needs. My heart pounds, and my palms sweat as I clutch the steering wheel. This is a toxic relationship. No one has to convince me of that. Yet, once more, I find myself entangled in his destructive world.

My plane lands. I walk outside of the Austin airport toward the curbside with my luggage in tow, and I see Dave standing there, leaning against his mother's white sports car. He looks every bit the part of a wealthy playboy, with his designer clothes and flashy jewelry. *He wears more jewelry than I do*, I think to myself. As he sees me approach, a grin spreads across his face, and he opens his arms for a hug. I smile back. I can't help but return the hug, even though I don't really want to. He pops the trunk of his car and puts my luggage in the back.

After leaving the airport, Dave recklessly steers onto a road he frequently favors. He loves this route for its particularly sharp turns and twists, broken up with occasional stretches of long highway. As usual, Dave puts his foot down on the accelerator and refuses to let up. My hand tightens on the door handle in the passenger seat, and my throat grows tight as I plead with him to slow down.

"Seriously? Shut the hell up. No one dictates how I drive!" Dave fires back sharply from the driver's seat. I sit motionless in the passenger seat, staring at the world zipping past my window. The speedometer moves steadily from 90 miles per hour to 100, then to 120, and finally creeps toward 130. My heartbeat matches the dizzying rhythm of the car's engine as the fields of central Texas blur into streaks of green and gold outside the window. My chest tightens with every second we accelerate.

As the car rockets forward, I can't help but reflect on the truth that love is blind, and it takes a while for the head and the heart to catch up. I know in my head this isn't right, but why don't I want to believe it? It's in that moment, as I am examining my lack of understanding of my own heart, that the real and honest truth hits me: I can't take it anymore. I glance to my left and see the speedometer vibrating near 130 miles per hour, and I make my decision. I am done with him. I can't risk telling him the truth just yet, but it's good enough for me to know. I just have to endure three more days with him, and then I will be on my way to the rest of my life, never looking back. Something inside me knows this decision is final. Even his magnetism is powerless against my resolve.

As we approach the final bend in a series of twists and turns, Dave, as always, relishes the chance to push the limits. I briefly wonder what his mom would think if she knew he was driving her brand-new car at such speeds. We veer right and then left, and that is the last thing I remember.

The story of what really happens that night remains a mystery. Dave's first recount of what causes the accident is that a deer suddenly leaps into our path, starting a chaotic dance of life, glass, and metal. Dave claims his natural response is to swerve in order to evade the inevitable collision with the animal, propelling our vehicle off the highway. According to expert investigation, it appears that the car soars into flight at such a height that its bottom grazes the top of a juvenile tree before smashing into a second, much larger one, bringing our frenzy to a halt.

The complete stop from such velocity is too powerful for any of the car's safety measures and my body hurls through the windshield into the night sky, landing me forty feet beyond the wreckage. Despite the totaled vehicle lying on the side of the road, my body vaults back onto the hard pavement, where I skid to a stop on a dashed yellow line in the middle of the interstate.

Witness to this chaos, a driver trailing closely behind us spun his vehicle around to see if he could help. The ultimate Good Samaritan, his heart urged him into the scene of an unfolding tragedy. He cautiously approached me as I lay, shattered, in the fetal position surrounded by a pool of blood and splintered glass. Just as he began to reach for his phone to call for an ambulance, a new horror was about to unfold—he could see a large semi-truck was heading in our direction. Careful not to move me to cause further injury, he acted on what can only be described as primal instinct, and sprinted toward the semi, frantically waving his arms high in the air to stop the truck from running over me. His panicked dance saved my life that night, diverting the truck's course away from my fragile body that had landed in the middle of the road. This Good Samaritan stood guard over me until paramedics arrived at the scene and took over.

The story goes that Dave emerged from the car, shaken, blood dripping from his forehead with a minor gash in need of a few stitches. Just as he began to process all that had transpired, he realized I was nowhere to be found. He frantically began searching for me. The car had landed far enough off the highway that it took him a couple of minutes to find me. Overwhelmed by a whirlwind of emotions, he was uncertain whether I was alive or dead, and knelt beside my broken body, which was desperately fighting to cling to life. "Caitlin, wake up! Wake up! Please, open your eyes!" Ever the one in charge, Dave ignored the warnings of the paramedics who had arrived on the scene, fearing that his actions of trying to move me would lead to further injuries. First responders began to carefully cut my clothing off as well as my boots, exposing a body lacerated with glass fragments from the windshield. One paramedic took note of a large piece of glass embedded in the right side of my leg. A doctor later said it was the largest piece of glass he had ever seen in one of his patients. During their thorough assessment of my body, I momentarily regained consciousness and with that a blood-curdling scream from the primal part of me that wanted to survive erupted out into the night.

It would be months after the accident, but I would eventually be given access to a police dash camera that captured footage from that life-changing night. The video is a chilling constellation made up of my horrifying screams and Dave's nonchalant chuckles. Just thinking about the way he jokingly described the accident to the police even now, sends a chill down my spine that overtakes my entire body.

As the head-to-toe examination continues in the midst of my painful cries, one of the paramedics makes a sobering observation: "It's rare to encounter a car ejection victim who is still alive," he says to his partner. In light of these statistics, survival is not in my favor. Paramedics know the situation is dire and carefully place my broken body onto a stretcher lifting me into an ambulance, heading to the nearest hospital, just five minutes away, so they could more thoroughly assess my injuries. There is no record of the man who came to my rescue that night. And I certainly can't recall his face. Yet, I hope, wherever he may be, somehow, he understands the depth of my gratitude.

My initial imaging workup reveals a severely shattered pelvis, as well as additional trauma throughout my body. Given that this was a small regional hospital, the medical team is not equipped to treat my life threatening injuries, so arrangements are made to transfer me via Life Flight to a hospital with a Level I trauma unit. However, due to extreme weather conditions a final decision is made by the medical team to transport me one and a half hours via ambulance instead. I was told this wasn't an easy decision because while there were many areas of concern, the major one was that I would lose too much blood and bleed to death from my injuries en route to the hospital. The ambulance driver knew this was an urgent mission and time was of the essence.

On the way to the hospital, EMT providers contact Summit Hospital to give them an estimated time of arrival so that they could prepare and activate a trauma team. The weather conditions are hazardous. It is dark. Heavy rains pour from the sky in sheets of water like it is monsoon season, reducing the ambulance driver's visibility. He has no other choice but to drive slowly and cautiously, intensifying the emergency as my body goes into cardiac arrest and flatlines. The paramedics jump into action, performing high-quality CPR on my lifeless body. Despite their efforts, I am without a pulse for several minutes. As challenging as it is to administer CPR during transport, they are successful in bringing me back to life.

When the ambulance arrives at Summit Hospital, I am whisked away to the emergency center. The team is a well-oiled machine, each member seamlessly performing their designated role. Nurses swiftly secure IV lines in my arms while monitoring my vital signs; others carefully examine the extent of my life threatening injuries. Amidst the controlled chaos, the lead surgeon discovers that my right leg no longer has a pulse, which puts me at high risk for a leg amputation. My leg had already been without a pulse for many hours, requiring the trauma team to move at warp speed with their assessment. Without any knowledge of my identity or history, the trauma surgeons begin making high-stakes decisions regarding my medical care. In most trauma fields there is what is referred to as the "golden hour"—the hour directly after injury when proper medical care is most likely to prevent death. I have far exceeded the golden hour, my situation beyond critical. It's for the surgeons to save my life now.

If I could hover over my own body to witness the chaos and confusion, I see bright lights causing my eyes to squint. An oxygen mask covers my nose, and a cervical collar around my neck prevents me from moving. Dozens of unfamiliar faces, covered by full-trauma protection gear, hover over me. I hear voices over the faint beeping of monitors, giving direct commands about my medical care. A nurse dressed in blue scrubs, a mask, hat, and gloves places her hand gently on my shoulder, offering me some comfort amid the tumult. "Can you tell me your name?" she asks gently. I try to move my mouth, but it is as if my body's ability to speak has been taken from me, along with everything else. I am in shock.

Just then, a man in the same standard blue medical uniform directs a question at me. "Ma'am, can you hear me? Open your eyes if you can hear me," he says. "You're going to feel several pokes; please do your best not to move." Only a local anesthetic is given—I feel several injections of lidocaine being pumped directly into my right thigh, just above the kneecap. The man works swiftly as he continues to stick me. Just when I think he is finished, I feel more painful pricks, and it takes me back to a memory when I am fifteen years old. I am staying at a friend's cabin, sleeping in a sleeping bag upstairs. Suddenly, I wake up to a sharp stinging sensation all over my knees. In a panic, I jump out of the sleeping bag and flip on the lights to discover a wasp nest inside, filled with angry wasps.

Another man appears, dressed head to toe in scrubs, and I see from the corner of my eye that he is holding a drill, much like what I could find in my dad's tool shed. A long rod is then attached to the end of the drill. I hear people talking frantically all around me. I take in the distressed looks on their faces as I register hands all over me. I panic as I realize I really cannot move. They are holding me down, but for what? The loud roar of the drill takes over my thoughts, and I cannot imagine a scenario where a tool like that would be used on a person who is still conscious. I want to scream, but it is impossible to find the words. *Don't they know I'm awake?* I am trapped in my worst nightmare. The rod, or what they call a "traction pin," is inserted straight through my right femur bone. In that moment, I don't know how the mind and body come together to endure the unendurable. I scream. I cry. I convulse. I hear the crunch of what sounds like bones being ground up, and I want to vomit. Those are my bones. And then the room goes dark.

I fade in and out of consciousness, experiencing a level of pain I didn't know was humanly possible. While I don't know it in this moment, the traumatic introduction to the ER is far from over. Weights are attached to opposite sides of the rod in my femur via a pulley system, and my left leg is yanked forcefully back into place to regain a pulse. The head of my femoral bone, forced out of its socket from the impact, has shoved directly into my pelvis, causing it to shatter. I remain in traction for the following three days while awaiting the arrival of a man who I later learn is one of the top orthopedic trauma surgeons in the country. Dr. Peter Anderson is out of the country when he gets the call regarding my injuries. The medical staff faxes over my X-rays for him to review. He informs his team to keep me stable until he returns to the States.

Later that evening, my parents receive a phone call that my mother can only describe as haunting. It is approaching midnight when my dad jolts upright out of bed at the sound of his phone ringing. He quickly answers, trying to shake himself awake. "Sir, your daughter is here at Summit Hospital in Texas. She was in a car accident," the operator says. My dad's heart rate spikes. "What's going on? What happened?" he asks. The operator responds calmly, "I'm sorry, sir. We cannot give you any information due to HIPAA regulations. I think it would be best for you and your wife to travel here immediately." My dad demands answers, but the operator calmly repeats his scripted responses about HIPAA violations. This leads my family to believe the accident isn't severe, thinking the gravity of the situation would surely have been communicated if it were that bad. Immediately, my parents and sister pack their bags and travel from Florida to Texas to be by my side.

When my parents rush into the hospital, leaving my sister in the waiting room, a trauma team descends upon them, bombarding them with detailed descriptions of my injuries and a laundry list of worst-case scenarios that could unfold. My dad later describes the moment as one of utter overwhelm and helplessness. As he processes what the doctors are saying, his chest tightens as the reality of my condition sets in. The scene at the hospital is chaotic and tense. The doctors and nurses speak a language my parents don't fully understand. Their medical jargon and terminology only add to the mounting fear that they are going to lose me—and to the confusion over why this happened in the first place.

My dad says my mom, though teary-eyed, remains stoic when they are escorted to the Level I trauma unit where I lie unconscious, lost in a haze of sedation. My mom hardly recognizes me, her middle child. My sister is in shock—she has just seen me the night before, all dressed up, makeup done, not a hair out of place. Now, my hair is a wild, tangled mess wrapped in tiny shards of glass. My face is covered in dried blood and last night's makeup. Glass of all shapes and sizes litters the floor of my hospital bed. My body is swollen and puffy. My eyes are nearly swollen shut, black and blue. My jaw, split in half during the accident, now looks crooked and disjointed. The right side of my face is completely shattered and bruised. A large white sheet hides the trauma to the lower half of the wreckage that is me.

While the last ten hours have been absolute torture, the worst is yet to come. Surviving flatlining in the ambulance, bone drilling, and indescribable pain is not the end. I still have to survive multiple surgeries, one of which will last sixteen hours, as well as the ever-present risk of bleeding to death. As the doctors lay out every possible worst-case scenario, including the very real possibility that I may die on the operating table, my parents are overwhelmed with shock as they attempt to process what has happened. It is explained to them that my body has already endured a massive amount of trauma, and now I must undergo a "second accident" to piece my body back together again. It is a real-life "Humpty Dumpty" story, and I am, unfortunately, the main character.

FOUR

FROG IN A BLENDER

D r. Anderson arrived at Summit Hospital three days after the accident. As my orthopedic trauma surgeon, he knew what I was beginning to suspect; my road to recovery would be grueling. In preparation for a long and arduous surgical procedure, he completed a thorough assessment of my injuries, seeking to understand what pressing needs would be addressed first. Later that evening, he met with my parents in the waiting area which had essentially become their new living arrangements.

Like any concerned father, my dad had a lot of questions for Dr. Anderson. He patiently took the time to answer them, trying to ease my parents' worries and frustrations. My dad asked if the surgery would be like a hip replacement, to which Dr. Anderson replied, "Not even close. A hip replacement is a walk in the park compared to what your daughter is about to endure. Mike, Caitlin's body is like a frog that was placed in a blender."

My dad stood speechless as he tried to process what the surgeon was trying to communicate to him. Although the analogy was grotesque, it ultimately helped my parents understand the gravity of the situation. Dr. Anderson went on to explain that he had performed thousands of pelvic reconstructive surgeries in his career, and I made his top twenty list of most severely injured patients. What an award! He also mentioned that there was a high probability my right leg would be paralyzed following the surgery. Nerve damage was simply unavoidable in order to properly repair and fuse the bones back together; even the slightest mistake could affect my chances of ever walking again. As my dad continued to talk with the doctor, he realized why Dr. Anderson was the best surgeon for the job.

Once all questions were answered, Dr. Anderson excused himself to go back and check on me, leaving my parents standing in the waiting room, silently numb with shock and worry.

My mom kept a detailed journal of the events each day, along with my progress. She was told that if I survived the surgeries, I would have very little memory of the weeks ahead of me.

Journal entry 1. We were finally able to meet with Cait's surgeon who will be performing her pelvic reconstructive surgery. We were told by multiple sources that he is one of the top orthopedic trauma surgeons in the country, and

now we know why Cait was sent here. The news
of her injuries hit us hard, but we have peace
knowing she is in good hands.

After a week of being in traction and heavily sedated while strapped to a hospital bed, the day of the surgery finally arrived. I was wheeled into the operating room surrounded by a team of top-tier healthcare professionals. Known for his strong faith and compassionate nature, Dr. Anderson always made it a point to lead a prayer over his patients before any procedure.

Journal entry 2. Peggy is one of the nurses
assigned to Cait's case. She has been a great
source of comfort to me throughout this entire
ordeal. The day after Cait's surgery, Peggy
shared with me that Dr. Anderson prayed in the
operating room before starting the surgery. She
said his prayer gave the trauma team a sense
of peace and reassurance before taking on
the daunting task of piecing Cait's pelvis back
together again.

My parents sit in matching blue recliners in the waiting room, anxiously awaiting updates on my procedure—my sister, who was still in high school, had been picked up by my aunt and taken back home to Florida. Minutes feel like hours as they both watch the clock positioned on the white wall in front of them. Surrounded by grieving families gives the room an ominous feeling. My mom later said she prayed on and off for sixteen hours. Her prayers were not just for my physical well-being, but also for the strength and guidance of the team who would be responsible for my care. A grieving family who had also been dealt a tragic blow sat directly next to my parents. Their teenage daughter was fighting for her life after being in a coma for several weeks following a car accident that mirrored my own.

The somber atmosphere in the room is palpable, and the silence is only broken by the occasional sound of someone stifling a sob. Suddenly, the door opens, and a lead surgeon enters the waiting area. My parents brace themselves, expecting the worst news about my own condition. But to their surprise, the surgeon makes his way to the family they had gotten acquainted with during their time in the waiting room.

The expression on the surgeon's face was grave as he delivered the devastating news that they would have to make the difficult decision to remove life support on their daughter that day. Up until that point, my mom had managed to hold herself together despite the overwhelming stress and worry. But as she watched the scene unfold in front of her, she couldn't contain her emotions any longer. She broke down, unable to imagine the pain and heartache that the other family was going through. She cried for that family and the unknown fate of her own child. The entire waiting area was now filled with a sense of shared grief and empathy.

My mom's heart went out to the family who had become a part of their lives in such a tragic circumstance. It was a stark reminder of the fragility of life and the unpredictable nature of accidents.

A long day and night laid ahead for the trauma team. Dr. Anderson worked tirelessly as he meticulously pieced my pelvis back together bone by bone. "It was like a puzzle," he remarked to someone, "trying to fit the pieces back together without disturbing the delicate balance." He cut through multiple nerves and layers upon layers of soft tissue. A staggering eighteen units of blood products were given. Later, I learned I flatlined twice during surgery. The first time I flatlined, the medical team quickly recognized the problem and sprang into action. Using advanced medical equipment and techniques, they were able to revive me and restore my heart's rhythm. But just when everyone thought the worst was over, I flatlined again. The second instance of flatlining was even scarier than the first. My body had already lost a significant amount of blood, and the odds were against me. But the doctors refused to give up, and they continued to work tirelessly to bring me back to life.

As the sun slowly descended, my mom began to nervously pace back and forth in the hospital waiting area. My dad, on the other hand, was struggling to keep his eyes open as he sat in his chair, his body succumbing to the physical and emotional exhaustion of the day. Just when my dad was about to doze off in his chair, Dr. Anderson entered through the double doors. He appeared tired but very pleased with his work. "I wanted to inform you that the surgery is over, and Caitlin is stable and in recovery," he whispered. As my parents beamed with relief, Dr. Anderson inquired about my home life. "Does Caitlin have a stable home to return to once she gets the green light from us?" My dad replied confidently, "Yes, she does. She will be well taken care of by her mother and me."

Dr. Anderson, being a seasoned surgeon, understood the importance of a stable home environment for a full recovery. He then explained to my parents the challenges I would face in the coming months—extreme pain and being confined to a hospital bed. Dr. Anderson could see the questions and worries in their eyes. "Please don't hesitate to ask any questions or voice any concerns you may have," he said, looking at my parents with compassion. "I want you to feel informed and involved in your daughter's care."

My parents nodded, grateful for a doctor who took time to listen and address their worries. In the end, many hands made sure the surgery was a success, and once again, I survived.

Dr. Anderson's words resonated with my family as I was wheeled into recovery, "It's going to be a long road, but she's a fighter. We've given her a chance."

The days in the trauma intensive care unit unfolded as a blur of discomfort and sporadic lucidity. Mom and Dad's voices remained a steady comfort and reminded me, "You've come so far. You're stronger than you know." The morning after my surgery, my parents were taken to the trauma ICU to see me post-surgery. They only had fifteen minutes with me. My mom was taken aback by my swollen body and hardly recognized me. Tears welled up in my parents' eyes as they softly spoke words of encouragement in my ear. In the following weeks, I was visited by friends and family who traveled long distances to be by my side. Although I have no memory of this, I am forever grateful for the immense support I received during my recovery.

Dr. Anderson's care and attention extended beyond just the surgery—he made sure my family and I were comforted and well-informed every step of the way. As the days dragged on, my body was consumed by a pain so intense that it defied all forms of measurement. With every breath, it felt like a thousand needles were piercing through my skin, tearing apart my insides. Despite being administered morphine and fentanyl around the clock, the excruciating agony remained unrelenting. As a result, I descended into a state of psychosis, a terrifying experience that I never could have imagined.

I am in a dark, eerie tunnel, with no recollection of how I got there. Panic sets in. My entire body goes numb, as if it is drained of all life. And then I notice something in the distance—a faint light flickering at the end of the tunnel. It is almost hypnotic, drawing me into its glow. At this moment, I feel a strange calm wash over me. It's as if my body is giving up, surrendering to the pain that is consuming me. The light offers a sense of comfort, a glimmer of hope in a terrifying ordeal. I continue to stare, and I can't help but wonder if I am dying. Is this the end of my suffering? Or is this something far more sinister, waiting to consume me completely? Even in my worst nightmare I could always wake up and escape. But this time, there is no waking up. I am trapped with no way out. For days on end, I am consumed by delusions, convinced that the people entering my room are strangers trying to kill me. I frantically seek refuge under my sheets, my mind consumed by fear and confusion. My mom describes my expression as that of a deer in the headlights, a look of pure terror permanently etched on my face. It feels like I have been plunged into a nightmarish world, a place that resembles hell itself. The physical pain may have been unbearable, but the mental anguish is equally torturous. I am trapped in a vicious cycle of hallucinations and paranoia, unable to distinguish reality from my distorted perceptions.

It is a strange and unsettling feeling to vividly recall my hallucinations. In one particularly horrifying episode, I wake up in the middle of the night to find spiders and roaches crawling everywhere, scurrying across the sheets and making their way onto my body. I am petrified and scream for help, desperate for someone to come to my rescue. In the midst of my panic, I notice my mom sitting in the corner of the room, studying me with a worried expression. I turn to her, desperate for an explanation as to why we were staying in such a filthy and unsanitary place. I tell her I am going to contact the head of the hospital and we are leaving immediately.

To my surprise, my mom laughs and replies, "That's my girl!"

While she is concerned that I am hallucinating, she is happy to see I have gotten my spunk back. I am taken aback and frustrated. How could she find this situation amusing? "Don't these people have any sense of cleanliness?" I demand.

It's then that I notice a woman with long, red hair standing in my doorway. She is heavily made up, a cigarette dangling from her fingers as she leans against the door frame. I stare at her, baffled and irritated. *Who is she? Why is she in my room?*

"Mom, who is this woman with the cigarette? I don't want to breathe in secondhand smoke," I shout, brushing at imaginary spiders crawling on my skin. My mom quickly reassures me there are no bugs, no rats, no creepy creatures, no woman with a cigarette—none of it is real. She tells me it's all a hallucination, a cruel trick of the morphine coursing through my body. I search her face, unsure if I can believe her. Fear, anger, and confusion flood my senses. It's so surreal, seeing things that aren't there.

"Why do I even need morphine? What's going on?" I demand, my voice trembling.

It's a long, restless night. The hallucinations refuse to let up. Bugs keep swarming over me, their phantom legs tickling my skin as I pick them off one by one and fling them across the room. My mom tries to comfort me, her soothing voice constant, but I keep insisting she's wrong—those bugs are real.

As the pain grows sharper, so does the dosage of morphine, and with it, the hallucinations intensify. Neither of us gets any sleep. One night, the pain is so unbearable it feels like my body is on fire. I start screaming, begging for help. The screams tear through my throat, louder and more desperate, until I rip the IV out of my arm. My mom is beside herself. She paces the halls, searching for a nurse.

But it's the weekend, and the hospital feels deserted. The halls are empty, silent, not a soul in sight. My mom later tells me how helpless she felt, standing outside my door, listening to my agonizing cries. Eventually, her composure crumbles, and she breaks down, crying too.

Finally, a nurse appears, hurrying through the double doors. She takes one look at my mom and calls my surgeon, who is on call that night. He arrives later, visibly upset when he learns how poorly my pain is being managed. My mom tells me afterward, "He had those nurses hopping!"

It turns out the nerves in my shattered pelvis are firing wildly, sending searing pain signals through my body. My surgeon prescribes a new medication specifically for this kind of pain. Slowly, the burning fire subsides, though the discomfort never truly leaves.

The sound of the door creaking open startles me awake. I groggily open my eyes, squinting against the harsh light of the room. I glance down at my arms, dark and mottled with black-and-blue bruises, each one a testament to the countless needle pricks I've endured. It feels like endless torture. My body is heavy, my limbs stiff from lying still for so long.

I don't know how long I've been asleep, but the darkness outside the window tells me it's the middle of the night. A male nurse approaches with a syringe in hand, his face somber, ready to administer the medication that keeps blood clots from forming while I'm immobile. Before I can even process what's happening, he lifts my hospital gown to expose my abdomen. I feel vulnerable, exposed, but I'm too tired to protest.

"Take a deep breath," he says. "This is going to be painful."

I close my eyes, bracing myself. The needle pierces my abdomen, sharp and stinging. Tears prick the corners of my eyes, but I refuse to let them fall. I don't want him to see me cry. As the liquid enters my body, I hear the clicking sound of the syringe. I focus on anything else—the sterile white walls, the beeping machines, the antiseptic smell—all of it feels foreign to me.

I'm young, vibrant. This kind of thing doesn't happen to people like me. But here I am, stuck in this hospital bed, enduring a never-ending cycle of pain.

Over the next ten days, visitors trickle in and out of my hospital room to see me, though I don't remember any of it. A constant supply of morphine flows into my body, managing the pain and keeping me comfortable, but it also conveniently keeps me unconscious.

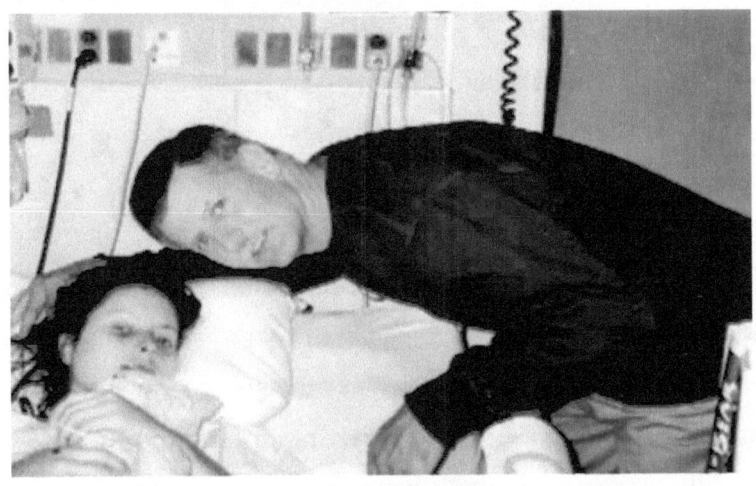

After two weeks confined to my bed, I am finally transferred to the intermediate ICU. On the morning of my move, a man in a white lab coat, his pockets full of pens and medical instruments, walks into my room. He has a strange familiarity about him. As he moves to the side of my bed, he smiles warmly, his expression radiating a genuine joy to see me awake. There's a brightness in his eyes, an energy that makes me feel calm and safe.

His eyes dart around the room, scanning the monitors, pausing in silent observation, and quickly processing the information they provide. I murmur through my wired-shut jaw, "Hi, I'm Caitlin. I was in a bad car accident, and my pelvis was shattered."

He smiles and responds with words that shock me. "I know. I'm the one who put you back together. It took sixteen hours, so we're well acquainted."

Suddenly, it clicks. This man standing in front of me is Dr. Anderson, the surgeon who saved my life. I can't believe I have no memory of him—a man so integral to my survival—but I know about him because of what my parents have told me. Tears well up in my eyes as I try to thank him, but the words won't come out. My wired jaw refuses to let me speak. I try again, struggling to form a simple "thank you," but the effort is futile.

Dr. Anderson smiles, his expression kind and understanding, and he pats my hand. "You don't have to say anything," he assures me. His warmth and reassurance put me at ease, the same way I imagine he did when I was on the brink of death. "You get some rest. I'll be back to check on you very soon," he says as he places my chart at the foot of the bed and leaves to see another patient.

Time in the hospital begins to blur. The hours stretch into days, and each one crawls at a snail's pace. My days are a haze of pain and medications, interrupted only by brief moments of consciousness. I stare at the ceiling, my thoughts disjointed and fragmented. Doctors and nurses come and go, offering bits of information I can't fully process. I catch fragments of their words, questions, updates, prognoses—but none of it feels real.

Despite my disoriented state, I am still acutely aware of time passing. I watch as the sunlight shifts through the window, casting shadows across the room. Day turns to night, and night back into day. The gentle rise and fall of my chest becomes the only reassurance I need: I am still alive.

Alive, yes, but trapped. Trapped in the waiting—waiting for my body to heal, waiting for my mind to awaken.

FIVE

COMING OUT OF THE FOG

Gradually, I emerge from my medicated slumber, but the cognizance of time eludes me. My hospital room has become a blur of memories, and I struggle to make sense of it all. Despite the consistent doses of morphine and fentanyl, for the first time since the accident happened, a heightened awareness envelops me, overtaking the hazy days that have preceded. The soft hum coming from a nurse along with the rhythmic click of her keyboard fills the room. I shift my gaze to find her immersed in her work at a desk in the corner of my room.

The weight of my cast, a pink plaster extending from my midthigh to foot, feels like an anvil that has been attached to my body in the form of my right leg. It is the first time I have truly noticed the discomfort it brings. *Did they apply it too tight?* I wonder as I stretch and try to find some relief by changing my position. No matter how I move, it feels like a boa constrictor is squeezing the life out of my leg. And the itching! It's like there is a host of fleas trying to dig at my skin. I miserably realize I'm too weak to even attempt to scratch.

My lips burn. Communication proves to be difficult with my mouth wired tightly shut. The young nurse, clad in pink scrubs, hair elegantly gathered in a low bun, rises from her chair and approaches me. Observing my chapped lips, she gives me a sympathetic smile as she acknowledges exactly what I am thinking: "Unfortunately, the morphine will do that." She exits the room for a moment and returns, holding a tube of chapstick, a soothing balm for my parched lips. The nurse gently separates my lips with her fingers, being careful not to disturb the wires embedded in my upper and lower gums that bind my mouth shut. She applies a thick coat of chapstick, and I feel immediate relief. The coolness of the balm soothes my burning lips.

I lie there still, but my mind is moving, as I attempt to reconstruct the fragments of my memory. As I try to mentally go from hopping into Dave's mother's sports car at the airport to the moment I regain consciousness in the trauma ICU, my mom quietly enters, taking her designated seat beside my hospital bed. In her journal entry for the day, she remarks that though I am conscious, I am still not "all there." She attributes that to the potent medications coursing through my veins. Repeatedly, I pose the same questions, striving to unravel the enigma surrounding me.

With each repetitive question I ask, patiently, my mother responds, "You were in a bad car accident, Cait. But you're still with us, and now your job is to rest and fully recover."

Concern for Dave enters my thoughts, even though he somehow walked away with only a small gash on his forehead. And strangely, I have no recollection of him visiting me in the trauma unit. I've been told that he did visit, but was only allowed short, ten-minute spurts. However, a fleeting memory of his parents making a brief appearance lingers. Though I can't recall details of the words exchanged, I vividly remember attempting to smile at Dave's father, exposing the wires in my mouth, as he observed me from across the hospital room. Even through the pain medication, I registered the sadness and concern on his face. I felt a strong need to somehow apologize for what had happened. Yes, it was Dave's fault that I was lying there, broken and bruised. But for some reason, I couldn't shake the urge to take responsibility for the accident and for the fact that his mother's car was now totaled.

"I'm sorry," I managed to say, the wires making it difficult to form words. My mom leaned in, her gentle touch on my shoulder, trying to make sense of my garbled speech. She soon realized the message I was trying to convey to Dave's father.

"It's okay, just rest," she said, her voice soothing and reassuring. My eyes closed as exhaustion took over, and my mom turned to face Dave's father. It was clear that he couldn't understand what I was trying to say.

Because of my mom's journaling during this time, I learn about this missing period of my life. Once she was informed by my surgeon that I wouldn't remember much of my time at the hospital, she kept a petite black journal and pen inside her purse, diligently recording the details of our journey. Most evenings she would sit by my bedside journaling about the events of the day, medications I was on, and cards and gifts we would receive. Mom, being an educator at a classical Christian school and having taught subjects such as English and Latin, was accustomed to journaling and creating schedules. It was a way for her to keep her notes organized, document my progress, and find a sense of control in a situation that was out of her hands.

Mom's journal entry. It's Tuesday morning. Due to the severe nature of Cait's injuries, she hasn't been allowed to shower. A couple of nurses entered our room and discussed cutting off Cait's hair. Her hair has become quite matted/knotted, and this seems to be the only solution. If I know Cait, she will absolutely object to this decision, so I am determined to comb every knot out of her hair. I am not sure if it can be done, and it will probably take days, but I am at least going to give it a solid effort.

Mom employed her schoolteacher mentality of determination and worked diligently as she began sectioning my long, thick hair and gently combed through the knots. She was right—it took three days, several styles of combs, hairbrushes, and leave-in conditioners, but she managed to untangle every single knot from my hair. Peggy, one of the lead nurses, told me weeks later that it was a true labor of love and it brought many of the nurses to tears, watching my mom gently pull through my bloody matted strands of hair as gently as if I were a child, just freshly showered, getting ready for bedtime. I was blown away by my mom's resolve and her decision to salvage my hair, despite the extreme hospital bed head.

The day my mom combed the final knot from my hair was also the day I was transferred to the rehab hospital—it felt like a double victory. I have no memory of this day, just a 5x7 photo of me, wheelchair bound, dressed in a bluish-green hospital gown with a single white compression stocking on my left leg, and a long, pink leg cast on my right side. I still have that same deer-in-the-headlights look on my face as I was wheeled by hospital staff to a rolling stretcher. It was as if life had been drained from my body and there was no vitality left. Whenever we recount this day, my parents remember how hopeful they were that I was going to continue healing.

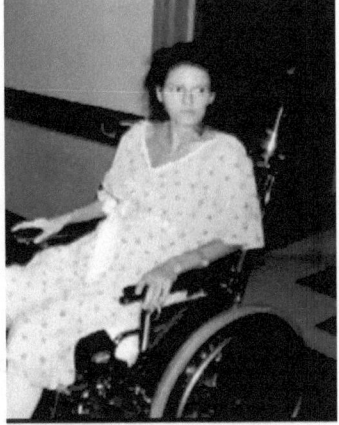

After enduring weeks of being confined to a hospital bed, my mind remained in a constant state of uncertainty as I drifted in and out of sleep. My body felt so incredibly weak, and at times, was reflected when I would fall asleep midsentence. I was still heavily medicated on morphine and fentanyl, as well as additional medications, but at some point, during my stay at the rehab facility, I finally emerged from the haze. Slowly I began to piece together the events of the situation that led me to this hospital bed.

I kept asking questions. I wanted to know details: *What caused our vehicle to crash? When do I get to go home? What is my long-term prognosis?*

Up until this point, my surgeon had kept the paralysis in my right leg from me. "Let's give it some time. I don't want to break her spirit," he told my mom.

Dave's visits to see me were infrequent and brief, but he appeared to be somewhat supportive. He would give my mom, who was staying with me to help take care of me, the occasional and much-needed break. However, it was evident, even to me, in my medicated and pain-filled state, that he was in denial about my condition. He treated me as though I had just suffered a minor athletic injury, rather than the severe trauma that I had actually survived.

I am on a strict, all-liquid diet, due to my mouth being wired shut, but Dave decides to bring in Max Muscle protein powder to "speed up my recovery." He places the black and red tub of protein powder onto the table. As soon as he lifts the lid and breaks the seal, the revolting smell of protein powder hits my nostrils. I turn my head in disgust, exchanging glances with my sister who is in town with my dad for a quick visit. My parents were out running errands, so it was just the four of us—my sister, Dave, me, and my nurse, who was quietly standing in the doorway. My sister had always been open about her dislike for Dave, and I could tell she was struggling to hold back her feelings at this moment.

"I don't think I can stomach that, Dave," I said, trying to decline his offer. But instead of respecting my decision, he responded sharply, "Do you want to get better? Do you want to get out of this hospital bed?" I was startled by his tone and before I could even respond, he continued, "You need to start taking action and actually doing something for a change." *Doing something? What does he mean by that? I can't do anything but lie here in this bed.*

I hated him. Every part of him. I picture myself breaking free of this hospital bed and tackling him to the ground. I can feel my sister's eyes on me, and I know she is wanting to speak up. She is so young, and I am sure Dave's intimidating presence is overwhelming for her. Looking back, she told me that it took every ounce of self-control not to go off on him, as she didn't want to cause a scene and create more stress for me. Even though Dave's presence alone was already accomplishing that.

Dave's well-intended gesture was also met with disapproval from one of the nurses who had grown fond of me during my stay. She couldn't hold back her feelings on the protein-powder matter and bluntly told Dave, "I don't think you understand what your girlfriend just went through. Her bones were shattered, and she nearly died." Her words were sharp and to the point, and it was clear that she was standing up for my well-being. She turned and winked at me. While I was grateful to have her in my corner, Dave, on the other hand, was taken aback and speechless. Ego bruised by the nurse's remarks, he didn't stay long that evening, and I was relieved as I watched him take his protein powder and head out the door. I started to notice that whenever Dave came to visit, my mom left the room, but a nurse would always be close by. It was evident that they did not trust him to be alone with me. This realization was disheartening, but it also made me appreciate the compassionate and watchful care of the nurses even more.

Overnight guests were not permitted at the rehab hospital, but an exception was made for my mom who would take over as my primary caretaker once I was released. Dave had booked himself a hotel room just days after the accident and that is where he remained for much of my stay at the rehab hospital. The day after the protein-powder incident, he popped in for another quick visit while my parents and sister were grabbing lunch. Dave sat in a chair next to my hospital bed as he devoured his meal from a "local gem" of a restaurant he discovered in downtown Dallas.

He dined his way through the city, dropping by the hospital to check on me from time to time. Every time he entered the room, he brought a bag of something mouthwatering to eat while I attempted to awkwardly drink a cup of pureed eggs through a straw from a tiny opening on the right side of my mouth. It was torture. I was so hungry and all I wanted was to be able to get up, walk across the hospital room, grab the burger from Dave's hands, and chomp down on the meaty goodness.

"What happened the night of the accident?" I asked him as he emptied a container of truffle fries and wiped the grease on a napkin. "Are you certain there was a deer? It just doesn't make sense to me that you even saw a deer if we were traveling at such a high rate of speed," I continued to press.

Dave always said the same thing, "It was a deer and that's all you need to know. I don't want to talk about it anymore,"

As I lay in this hospital bed, a part of me couldn't shake the feeling that he was lying about the events that led to my current state. But I was too tired to push the matter and always changed the subject. Communication was a challenge for me, I struggled to speak because of the wires binding my mouth shut and the overwhelming fatigue from the trauma I had experienced. Dave finished his lunch and patted my shoulder, before making his way toward the door. "I'll be back tomorrow," he said as he turned to leave. I simply nodded, too drained to even form a response, and closed my eyes in hopes of finding some rest. Finally, he was gone, and I could escape into sleep.

But I couldn't sleep. It was hard for me to trust his words and actions, especially after what had happened. While the accident had left me physically broken, it had also left me with a shattered sense of trust. I knew he was keeping something from me. Dave had a history of telling little white lies. His ability to deceive was uncanny, and I had caught him in the act on several occasions. He also seemed to have no qualms about lying to his own parents, as if it were second nature to him. As I lay awake, my mind raced with thoughts of what he could be hiding from me. *Was he under the influence when he picked me up from the airport? Did he receive a drug test?*

From a young age, I was always praised by my dad for my street smarts. He compared me to a private investigator—able to unravel any mystery and not easily swayed by deception. *Soon*, I thought. *When I am feeling stronger, I will confront him and get to the bottom of this.*

*   *   *

Every morning, I would dread opening my eyes. Pain had become my new alarm clock. The feeling that I was on fire would jolt me out of sleep first thing in the morning. My body would be engulfed by excruciating pain; it felt like open sores on the lower half of my body. The once peaceful act of sleeping had become a source of agony for me. The pain was a constant companion, never leaving me—even for a moment. My back and neck were particularly affected, muscles and ligaments had been ripped and torn from the places in my body where they belonged. Inflammation, causing my back to swell, made it difficult for me to move. I was constantly rotating between ice packs and heating pads, searching for relief. But the discomfort was inescapable as I was forced to lie flat on my back, unable to shift to either side, the pressure on my nerve endings causing an intense burning sensation everywhere. Yet the hospital bed I was confined to had a sign hanging above it with a warning: "Do not rotate patient on left or right side. Patient must lie on her back at all times." This only added to the agony I faced.

I was struggling both physically and mentally. It was a constant battle. I started to experience high blood pressure due to the stress and strain on my body. My doctor prescribed a medication to control it, adding to the ever-growing list of pills I was already taking.

* * *

As I step into the steamy shower, the warm water cascading down my body is a familiar and comforting feeling, and I luxuriate in the act of getting clean. On the other side of the shower door, I can hear the beeping of my coffee pot, but want to linger a little longer. I step out of my shower, taking long deep breaths, slide into warm, fuzzy slippers, and take in the aroma of freshly brewed coffee. All of my senses are awakened as I make my way to the kitchen. The beeping of the coffee maker interrupts my blissful thoughts. I open my eyes and am struck with the realization that the beeping is not coming from my coffee pot, but from a monitor next to my bed. Instead of fuzzy slippers on my feet, I have a full length leg cast on my right leg and a compression sock on my left. I struggle in my confusion. It was all so real. The refreshing, hot shower, the smell of the coffee. Tears slide down the sides of each eye, into my matted hair as I continue to listen to the beeping of the monitor I am tied to. It's a constant reminder of the reality I face every day. Gone are the simple pleasures of a warm shower and a cup of coffee. I wonder if I will ever see them again. Instead, my mornings now begin with a Fragmin shot in the stomach to prevent blood clots and a pureed beverage for breakfast. I quickly learned you could puree just about anything. A brown liquid substance of hamburger and egg often made it on my food tray. I reached a point where I couldn't stomach it any longer and started requesting only chicken broth and chocolate Ensures. It was at least palatable and provided me with some nutrients.

*   *   *

"Today's the day!" my mom sang out cheerfully, pulling back the curtains and allowing the warm rays of sunshine to filter into my new living space at the rehabilitation hospital. I so appreciated the small glimpse of the outside world that the window provided me.

"While you were sleeping, I heard one of the nurses mention that you'll be getting your first bath today!" my mom continued, still with that same cheerful and excited tone.

A bath, I thought to myself, *that sounds amazing*. I couldn't recall the last time I had taken a proper bath, and with the constant sweating caused by my medications, I was in desperate need of some cleanliness.

"It's bath time!" one of the nurses announced with a smile as she enters the room. I had been so fixated on the final outcome of feeling clean, that it suddenly dawned on me that I had no idea how they would actually get me into a bathtub. I could barely make it to a wheelchair. Sensing my concern, the nurse reassured me, "Don't worry, this will be a bed bath. We'll guide you through the process, and you'll feel clean and refreshed in no time."

A bed bath? I blinked back tears of disappointment as my heart sank. I wouldn't be getting the luxurious soak in a bathtub that I had been daydreaming about. I knew I didn't have a choice because I was filthy and in desperate need of a good scrubbing, so I had to accept it.

"We're going to gently place this waterproof cover underneath you," the nurse explained, emphasizing the word gently. She and her colleague carefully maneuvered the cover under my body, making sure to cover every inch of my back. I was still wearing my hospital gown as they worked.

"I'll need to remove your gown and cover you with this sheet," the nurse went on to tell me. Her colleague had left the room to fill a basin with warm water, and when she returned, they both lathered the rags with foamy soap and began bathing me. It was a humbling experience to say the least.

As they washed me from head to toe, I couldn't help but feel a confusing mix of embarrassment and gratitude. On one hand, I was embarrassed because it was personal and intrusive, but on the other hand, I was grateful for the care and compassion of the nurses. I started to shiver as the water dripped off me onto the plastic-like cover. After all the body parts that they could get to had been washed, the final part to clean was my hair. I was grateful, once again, to my mom for committing to brushing it as they got busy lathering it with soap and pouring water over my head. It felt like an eternity, but finally, they were done. As if I were a newborn, they dressed me in a fresh gown, combed my hair, and tucked me into fresh bedding. It had been uncomfortable, but it was worth it. I was finally clean, the first time since the accident.

*   *   *

As I settle into a daily routine at the rehabilitation hospital, I can't help but feel overwhelmed by a sense of monotony that causes frustration. It's all the same.

Wake up because my body feels like it's on fire.

Medications and Ensure drink.

Fragmin shot in the stomach.

Physical therapy.

As I slowly sip the last few drops of my Ensure drink through a small gap between my teeth, I take a deep breath, mustering the strength to tackle the day. I am wheeled down the hallway toward the rehabilitation room, and I take in my surroundings. Now that I am more aware, I notice the other injured patients around me, and I wonder about the extent of their injuries and how long they have been here. Some of them look like they've been here for a long time.

While I am moved from my wheelchair to a wooden table, I wonder if that is going to be me. *I won't let that be me.* My resolve to be the best patient so I can get out of here propels me to endure the discomfort of pressure on my tailbone while on the table. As the session begins, I fight to stay awake from the pain medications and morphine as the therapists, on either side of me, slowly lift my legs one at a time. Upon waking, I can't help but feel discouraged. *Is this all there is?* I think to myself. I know deep down that I am capable of so much more. All I have done is switch from lying in a hospital bed to lying on a therapy table. I search for a way to identify how I'm feeling and realize, for the first time, I am feeling angry. I am angry at myself. *I put myself here*, I keep thinking. *This is my fault. I knew I should never have gotten into the car with him.* My mind begins to seethe as I am transferred from the table back into the wheelchair. I am angry that my once strong body is now frail and weak. I am angry that I have to live in this hospital. I am angry that I have to drink liquified scrambled eggs every morning. I try, but I can't stop the tears from flowing. They come in waves as grief over everything I have lost takes over my body. My mom, who has been there the whole time, is at a loss for words. I hate crying in front of other people, especially people I don't know. The therapists look at each other and step away to give me a moment with my mom.

"I have to get out of here," I sob, taking long drags of air.

"We can't leave until your surgeon gives us the green light, Cait. You know that," my mom replies in a soft voice, trying to comfort me.

I sob even harder remembering she has made arrangements with her work to take a year off to serve as my primary caretaker here in the hospital, and then once I return home. I swallow hard and take in a deep breath as I wipe my tears. Each time I begin to feel sadness over my situation that day, I try to compartmentalize my thoughts. *Just don't think about anything*, I would tell myself. But it was hard not to think about everything that had led me to this moment.

One by one, I would recount the events that brought me here. The accident, Dave, my injuries and surgeries. It was overwhelming and I felt frustrated and defeated.

As I lay on the therapy table, a sense of defeat washes over me, threatening to drown me. It's just more lying down and more leg lifting—how is any of this ever going to make a difference? As my nurse wheels me back to my room, I begin questioning her.

"What do I need to do in order to return home?" I watch her like a hawk, not wanting to miss any cues or reactions. "Is there any way you can give me a list? Things I can do and check them off as I accomplish them?" Even as a child, I was always a list maker. I remember in elementary school writing out a to-do list each week and feeling a sense of accomplishment as I completed each task. I needed something to work toward and crossing things off a list gave me a much-needed sense of accomplishment. The nurse looked a bit perplexed as she considered my request, but I was determined. I would do whatever I needed to do to get home.

"I am just so ready to get home," I explained as I looked her directly in the eye. Even with all the medication hampering my ability to communicate, I was desperately hoping she understood my urgency. Thankfully, she nodded and answered quickly. "I can make a list for you, if you'd like." My eyes lit up and my heart skipped a beat. Something to do, something to work toward, something to think about other than the how, what, where, when, and whys of how I ended up here in the first place.

"That would be great, thank you," I replied gratefully, as the nurse lifted me from the wheelchair and placed me back in my hospital bed.

Later that afternoon, I woke up from a nap and noticed a list on my food table. The nurse had been so kind to type up everything I needed to do, even categorizing it into basic physical therapy and occupational therapy, as well as additional tasks my mom would need to perform. "Mother will be required to continue with administering shots in the stomach until patient is mobile," I read aloud, feeling queasy at the thought. My mom was not going to like this.

The next morning, as the nurse entered with the dreaded shot, I spoke up. "Wait. Mom, I want you to do it." I could see the blood drain from my mother's face and the look of terror in her eyes. "I don't know if I can," she said in a quavering voice, her weak stomach when it came to anything medically related was always a joke in our family. After the accident, this was her worst nightmare. "Don't tell me that," I shook my head, determined to have her by my side. "I need you to do this, Mom. It's one step closer to home. And I need to go home." I watched as the nurse gave her a quick tutorial and handed her the shot. "You got this, Mom!" I encouraged. Reluctantly, she grabbed the shot and placed it over my abdomen. I watched her close her eyes and wince as she administered the injection into the soft tissue of my belly. I tensed up, waiting to hear the click and feel the shot roll out of her hands. She fumbled around, trying to grab it, and then stabbed me in the stomach. We both heard the click, and it was over.

"That wasn't so bad!" she exclaimed, relieved.

It hurt like hell, but I couldn't bring myself to tell her that. I was proud of her for facing her fears to help me get better. It was just one more thing to check off the list toward my ultimate goal—going home.

As the days went by in the hospital, I was overwhelmed with the love and outpouring of support from friends and family. Care packages filled with thoughtful items arrived at my bedside, along with countless letters and gifts from total strangers. It was a heartwarming reminder of the incredible community I had back home. They were rooting for me, and that felt really good.

One evening, my mom walked into my hospital room and handed me a letter. I pressed the incline button on my bed, lifting myself into an upright position, and eagerly began to open it. To my surprise, it was a three-page handwritten letter from someone I had always admired in high school who had been a few grades ahead of me. As I read through her carefully crafted words, tears streamed down my face. She was the same ole good-hearted Kensie I had always loved and respected. Kensie possessed a rare quality of selflessness, always going above and beyond with her support for those around her. Her nonjudgmental nature was a breath of fresh air—especially back in high school when our peers were quick to criticize. Her letter was a true reflection of her unwavering support and care for those around her.

* * *

I often found myself staring at the clock, wishing time would pass more quickly. But there was one thing that always brightened my week—a visit from Max, the hospital therapy dog. He was a beautiful, blonde golden retriever, and as he made his way to my bedside, I reached out to pet him, feeling the softness of his fur and the warmth of his body against my hand. He would then gently rest his head on the edge of my bed, as if he knew that was exactly where I needed him to be. Max's presence was always so comforting and reassuring, and I was grateful for his visits. On one particular day as Max was leaving my room, I turned to my mom and said, "Well, there's another thing I can add to my bucket list—get a golden retriever." My mom chuckled and replied, "I have no doubt that you will someday."

I finally graduated from the table exercises at therapy to being able to perform small movements with my legs in my wheelchair. I still had no use of my right leg, so I had to have a bit of help. The movements were small—up an inch, down an inch. There was also a contraption that I used to move my arms to help strengthen them. Some days we would play games like tic-tac-toe. At first, I wasn't sure what good these exercises were doing, but I was compliant and happy to at least be doing something seemingly productive.

I suppose some of the exercises were just meant to pass the time, or maybe they were testing to see if the concussion affected my memory. I wasn't quite sure, but one thing I did know was that I was willing to do anything to get out of that hospital room.

As I sit in my wheelchair, idly manipulating the game pieces in my hands, I am suddenly transported back to a distant time when I was a member of a flag football team. My dad was the coach, who possessed a vast repertoire of intricate and cunning trick plays. It was game day and our team was in the lead. My dad gave us the signal to perform the well-rehearsed trick play.

Without hesitation, we were in formation. As the ball snapped, my friend, a formidable quarterback, and I sprinted toward each other with a fervent determination. However, instead of a successful handoff, our foreheads collided, causing us to career backwards and land flat on our backs on the unforgiving grass. The impact of the collision gave us both mild concussions, leaving us each with a throbbing headache.

My reminiscence is abruptly cut short by the gentle touch of my nurse, who has arrived to escort me back to my room.

Even the simplest of outings would exhaust me—therapy sessions, a wheelchair ride around the hospital, or a trip to the food court. I felt drained. Despite the exhaustion, I was determined to push through and make progress. I believed these small movements and exercises were essential for my recovery, but I also longed for more significant progress. I wanted to be able to walk again and get back to my normal life. I missed going for runs around my neighborhood, dancing with my friends, and simply being able to move freely without any assistance. I knew I had to be patient, but unfortunately, patience has never been my strong suit.

Weekends were always the toughest for me. As a patient in the hospital, I dreaded them because most of the staff would leave and there would be no therapy sessions. Dave also left, his visits confined to a few days in the week and then back to his parents' home for the weekend. It felt like time was moving at a snail's pace, and I was stuck in this hospital room with nothing to do. My mom would try to keep me entertained by finding shows for us to watch on the television, but I couldn't stand the noise for too long. It was like every sound was amplified, and it was overwhelming. This sensitivity to lights and sounds was all new to me, something I had never experienced before.

One of the popular shows at the time was *Lost*, and I had watched a few episodes before my accident. My mom and I tried to catch up on the series, but I couldn't keep up with the fast paced storyline. It was too much for me to handle, and I would often end up putting a pillow over my head and plugging my ears to block out the noise. I couldn't help but wonder, if anything was ever going to be normal again. *What was wrong with me? Why was I suddenly so sensitive to sound and light?*

As each new Monday morning arrived, I would be overcome with a sense of relief. It meant I would finally be leaving the rehab hospital and heading to the actual hospital for my X-rays. It was a small moment of freedom from the constant confinement I had been experiencing.

My mom came in with my handheld mirror and toiletry bag. I used cotton pads and witch hazel to clean my skin, and then applied some lotion to my face. I pulled my greasy hair up into a high bun, trying to make myself look presentable. I then pulled out my toothbrush and mom sat a small bowl of water on my food tray.

I had a small, soft child-size toothbrush for the wires in my mouth, and I could only brush the front part of my teeth. Working for a dentist in the past, I knew the importance of frequent teeth brushing, and it was something I was always very meticulous about. But now, with the wires in my mouth, it made brushing difficult.

It was a small thing, but it bothered me greatly. My mom handed me a paper cup of bright blue mouthwash with a plastic straw. I swished it around in my mouth and then held the cup under my chin and over my food table to allow it to drain through the wires and back into the cup. I glanced into the handheld mirror once more and stared at my reflection for a bit longer than usual. My face looked thin and tired, cheeks sunken. I lifted my lips to reveal the silver wires binding my mouth shut. I didn't recognize myself. *Who was this girl looking back at me?*

As I lay in my hospital bed, I heard a cheerful humming enter my room. The door opened and in walked Dr. Anderson's medical assistant, a tall and strong-looking man with an infectious energy. "Hey little mama!" he greeted me with a warm smile. I awkwardly smiled back. I immediately liked him. He effortlessly lifted me off the bed as if I was a feather. "You don't weigh nothing!" he exclaimed with a chuckle. "What are they feeding you here?" I pointed to the wires in my mouth as I attempted to explain. "Oh goodness!" he said, still grinning. "Let's get you to the X-ray room."

He wheeled me across the bridge to Summit Hospital and into the X-ray room. To my surprise, Dr. Anderson was already there. "How's my favorite patient?" he greeted me with a big smile. "I am doing good, all things considered," I replied. "I am struggling a bit mentally though. My life revolved around physical activity, and now I'm forced to lie in the same position all day."

"I am sorry," he seemed genuinely empathetic. "With the exception of pain, the down time is going to be the toughest part." I sighed.

"Don't let it get the best of you," he encouraged me. "You are strong and the fact that you are young will aid in your recovery."

"Keep your head up, little mama!" his MA encouraged. We exchanged a fist bump before he lifted me onto the X-ray table. My pain medications were doubled that morning to get me through the process. As my body made contact with the cold, metal X-ray table, it seemed as if all my bones were exposed. The pain was terrible. Up until that point, I had not been conscious during these procedures. I gritted my teeth underneath the wires. Dr. Anderson's MA held my hand throughout the entire process. The pain was so intense, I started to sweat. Just when I thought I couldn't take it any longer, he lifted me from the table and placed me back in my wheelchair. "All done!" he said as I slumped over in my wheelchair, exhausted from pain. "Get the rolling stretcher," Dr. Anderson said. "I don't think she's going to tolerate the wheelchair for the ride back."

*　　*　　*

"I need to get out of here," I sobbed as tears fell from my cheeks. I slowly sipped a chocolate Ensure, feeling the weight of all my emotions take over me. My mom got up from her usual perch beside my bed and began to rub my head. It was the only time I felt the slightest bit relaxed.

"We can't rush this process," my mom explained for the hundredth time. She was only trying to comfort me, but I protested. "We can just leave, and you can continue with my care at home. I don't understand why we can't do that? I have already been here for three weeks. I'm losing my mind staring at these walls. I can't walk, I can't even rotate myself in this bed. I'm over it all."

"I know you are," my mom replied, her hand still gently rubbing my head. "But let's just give it a little longer. You haven't even started occupational therapy yet. Once you master that, let's reevaluate."

And so, the following week, I began occupational therapy. This type of therapy was designed to help me overcome my limitations due to my injuries as well as to help me live as independently as possible. Throughout this process, I was closely monitored by a team of occupational therapists.

As I stepped into the therapy center, my eyes were immediately drawn to the vast space filled with natural light pouring in from the large windows. My gaze then shifted to the various therapy stations scattered around the room where patients with varying degrees of ability were working on their exercises. I felt lost. Like I didn't belong here. This was a place I never thought I would find myself in. After all, I am young and vibrant, this kind of thing doesn't happen to someone like me.

But here I was, surrounded by individuals who were all facing their own physical challenges. As I observed them, I couldn't help but feel a sense of admiration for their determination and perseverance. Some were in wheelchairs performing slow and controlled mobility exercises, while others were lying on therapy tables. It was evident that we were all here for a common purpose—to heal and regain our independence.

As I made my way further into the room, I still couldn't shake off the feeling of being out of place. I had never been one to shy away from physical activity, and the thought of needing therapy to regain my strength was foreign to me. But the accident had left its mark on me, both physically and emotionally. And now, I had no choice but to face it head on.

I was wheeled to the back right corner of the room where I noticed a white simulator car. My mom and I exchanged glances, both confused as to why there was a car in the therapy center.

"Today, we are going to teach you and your mom how to properly transfer you from a wheelchair to a car." This was such a crucial skill for me to learn in order to regain my independence. My mom put on a brave face as she wheeled me as close to the passenger side door as possible. I gripped the handles of my wheelchair tightly as she carefully helped me lift my left leg into the car. Then, I slowly moved my right leg over to join my left. With my mom's assistance, I lifted my body into the car. It took a lot of effort, but I didn't give up. I just kept telling myself to do the next thing. The process of getting back into my wheelchair was just as difficult. Every movement was painful, but I closed my eyes and took deep breaths to better tolerate the pain.

Just do the next thing on the list, Caitlin.

First move the right leg.

Then move the left.

Use your arms to settle yourself into the seat.

It took a few days, but I eventually mastered the art of getting into a car, and my mom could transfer me safely from my hospital bed to the wheelchair independently. It was a huge achievement and one that filled me with a sense of pride and accomplishment. I also had my first shower using a shower bench, and it was a glorious experience. Despite my initial hesitation, the hot water running down my body felt like heaven, and it provided some much needed relief for my aching body. My mom was now able to assist me with showering and getting dressed, and I no longer had to wear a hospital gown. I was finally able to wear soft, loose clothing, although the pants were a few sizes too big to fit over my cast. But I didn't mind. It felt amazing to be wearing regular clothing again. It's the little things.

As another week passed by, I anxiously awaited Dr. Anderson's arrival in my hospital room. I could hear his familiar knock on the door and my heart raced with anticipation. He walked in with a warm smile, asking, "How are you doing today?" he made eye contact before going through my charts.

"I'm a bit stir-crazy, but I feel like I am well enough to go home," I answered.

Dr. Anderson's expression changed to one of surprise as he surveyed the state I was still in. "Let's not rush things," he replied, "Slow and steady wins the race. This is a *tough* injury to overcome."

He went on to explain that there are different degrees of pelvic injuries, some of which don't even require surgery. Unfortunately, mine was one of the worst he had seen in his professional career. But he promised that we would get me out of the hospital when the time was right. He praised my progress in therapy, saying that I was accomplishing things at a faster pace than anticipated.

"Let's talk in a week and we'll see about setting a release date," he said with a reassuring smile. Turning to my mom, he added, "Hang in there. I hear you are going to win the Mother of the Year award!" Her face lit up with gratitude and relief. I could see that she had been growing weary as well.

The next week dragged on painfully slowly. Each day was a mix of medications, pain, confinement, therapy, and restlessness. But I kept pushing through, knowing that each day was one step closer to going home.

Finally, Friday morning arrived, and I was sent in for X-rays again. Dr. Anderson asked my mom and his MA to accompany me. Thankfully, my X-rays looked great. Dr. Anderson sat in his chair as I faced him in my wheelchair. "Let's take a look at your incision."

I nervously lifted my hospital gown to reveal the scar from my pelvic reconstructive surgery. It was over a foot long and wrapped around my midsection and part of my back. But to my relief, Dr. Anderson smacked his lips in satisfaction, "It's healing very nicely. The stitches will eventually dissolve on their own, so there will be no need to remove them."

"Can you tell me about your home life?" Dr. Anderson inquired for a second time. Just as I was about to respond, an image of the female patient down the hall, who was around my age and had suffered similar injuries, entered my mind. She was sent to live in a nursing home for nine months due to not having a family to care for her. A sadness came over me, but I quickly redirected my thoughts to Dr. Anderson's question.

"Well, it's pretty normal," I replied. "My parents are great, as you can see, and I have two siblings. One is still at home and the other is away at college."

Dr. Anderson explained that he just wanted to make sure I had a stable environment to return to for my recovery. I reassured him that I had a loving and supportive family and friends who had already shown me immense support during my time in the hospital. He nodded and then proceeded to lay out what I could expect when I returned home. Since I would be living with my parents during my recovery, we would need to make some modifications to accommodate my wheelchair. This included installing a wheelchair ramp, a hospital bed, shower bench, toilet seat, and walker.

He also mentioned that he would personally choose a trauma surgeon in our area for me to see once a month for X-rays and monitoring. This was something he was very particular about. "It has to be an orthopedic *trauma* surgeon," he emphasized. "And I would prefer someone I know personally, even if it means driving a distance."

My mom would also have to arrange for in-home healthcare, with a nurse coming once a day and a physical therapist three times a week. I would be going home with a fentanyl pain patch, which could be dangerous if not used properly, and my mom would receive strict instructions on its usage. We were also told we needed to figure out a way to transport me to my parents' home in Florida. My options were a medical flight or an ambulance ride.

"A week from today!" Dr. Anderson said enthusiastically. "I'll perform my final evaluation and barring no complications between now and then, you are free to go," he said with a warm smile.

The idea of going home gave a glimmer of hope. As I adjusted my hospital bed upright and reached for my calendar, I marked "home" on the day a week away. "I am going home," I whispered to myself, as a wave of relief washed over me.

I had survived. And I was going home.

SIX

REALITY CHECK

I lie still on the hospital bed, staring at the ceiling. Tomorrow, I'm supposed to leave, heading home with my mom and a team of paramedics. Two months here, and I'm not even sure I remember what home feels like. The thought of leaving should fill me with relief, but it doesn't. My chest feels tight, my stomach heavy with dread. *What if something goes wrong? What if I'm not ready?* The questions loop endlessly, each one building on the next until I feel like I might scream.

The urge to move is unbearable. My body feels like it's encased in cement, and my mind won't stop screaming at it to do something—anything. My muscles feel locked, stiff and aching, as if every fiber of me is itching to stretch, to break free from this prison of stillness. The sensation is maddening. I want to sit up, swing my legs off the bed, pace the room just to prove I can. But I can't. The last time I tried something as simple as stretching in bed, it felt like my pelvis would rip in half, the pain so sharp and immediate it stole my breath. It left me terrified of trying again, yet the need to move hasn't gone away. If anything, it's worse now, a constant buzz of frustration under my skin. I press my palms against the sheets, trying to push through it, but it only makes me feel more trapped.

I grab the notepad and pencil a friend brought me. My hands are shaky, but I need to focus on something. Anything. I start sketching the window across the room. It's something to do, a poor substitute for what I really want—to stand, to walk, to feel alive in my body again. Drawing feels strange, like using a part of me that's been dormant too long, but I keep going, tracing the edges of the glass, the faint streaks of rain, the gray sky beyond. It's enough to dull the frustration, if only a little.

The door opens, and Dr. Anderson steps in with two nurses. "Hello," he says, his voice calm and steady. "Tomorrow's the big day, isn't it?"

I nod, gripping the pencil tighter. *Yes. Tomorrow.*

I make sure they know how very grateful I am to all the staff for the care I have received.

Dr. Anderson's reassuring smile offers a glimmer of comfort amidst the sea of uncertainty that surrounds me. His nod signals the beginning of yet another evaluation, a ritual that has become all too familiar during my stay in this hospital room.

As he directs his attention toward the incision that snakes its way across my midsection and back, I feel a surge of apprehension. I look away. "It's over a foot long," Dr. Anderson observes. My eyes dart back to the incision. The sight of the dark hues of purple and red on my skin makes my stomach churn. To look at it is to confront the raw reality of the fact that my abdomen was once wide-open exposing all of my organs. It's more than I can comprehend. I try to distract myself as he continues with the evaluation.

"Your incision continues to heal nicely," Dr. Anderson remarked, gently brushing his fingertips over the area. "The stitches will soon dissolve on their own, so there's no need for removal, as I mentioned previously." Even though I've heard this before, I still feel relief. *At last, a part of this recovery sounds manageable*, I think to myself.

And just like that, we transition to the next phase of the evaluation—a series of tasks designed to test my newfound capabilities. I look over to my mom for reassurance, breathing a grateful prayer for her steadfast support.

Together, we navigate the intricacies of transferring from bed to wheelchair, a delicate balance of coordination and cooperation. It's a process that demands patience, a quality I've never been known to possess in abundance. As I wrestle with the slow pace of rehabilitation, my mind drifts back to the echoes of my childhood, where every task was a battle against time itself. A perfectionist by nature, I approached each undertaking with a fervent need for speed and precision, driven by the desire to swiftly check it off my ever-expanding to-do list. My grandfather, a seasoned military man, was a master of organization. His meticulously crafted to-do lists adorned the walls of his home, serving as a constant reminder of the importance of order.

But faced with the daunting reality of my recovery, I was forced to confront a harsh truth: No amount of planning or list making could accelerate the healing process. It's a humbling realization, a bitter pill to swallow as I grapple with the limitations of my own nature. In this crucible of introspection, I find myself at a crossroads, tasked with embracing the slow, arduous journey toward healing.

With a thumbs up and a smile of approval, Dr. Anderson offers his final verdict, with a reminder to tread cautiously. "Two years before a semblance of normalcy will return," he says—a timeline that feels so overwhelming and distant, I can't quite wrap my head around it. But as I contemplate the road ahead, I refuse to let my mind wander too far into the future. The weight of it is too much for my battered body to carry.

"Let's have a little chat," Dr. Anderson looks at me, and then my mom, and my heart drops. I know immediately by his tone that this is not going to be a casual conversation. My mom moves her chair even closer to be next to me, as if trying to provide some comfort. I get the sense they all know something I don't know.

"What's going on?" I ask, my voice trembling with worry. "I am still going home tomorrow, right?" I try to sound nonchalant, but the fear in my voice was evident.

"Yes, you are," Dr. Anderson replies, trying to reassure me. "But I want to talk with you about your right leg. Have you noticed any sensation return? Can you wiggle your toes?" he asks, as he begins to examine my leg, again.

"I feel a constant burning pain and numbness from my toes to my midthigh," I reply. I try to wiggle my toes, to show him, but I can't. It feels as if my leg is detached from my body, and someone has superglued it back into place. Dr. Anderson nods, as if he expected that answer.

"I am sure it will get better as time progresses, right?" I ask, subconsciously begging him to agree with me.

"That's what I wanted to talk to you about," Dr. Anderson replies in a somber voice. "You see, during the pelvic reconstructive surgery, there was an extensive amount of nerve damage that we couldn't repair. I am sorry to have to tell you this, Cait, but your right leg is now paralyzed from the thigh down."

My heart sinks as the word *paralyzed* bounces off my brain. I can't believe what I am hearing. I want to put my hands over my ears and scream to drown out the words that are coming from his mouth. My mind races, struggling to process this unwelcome update, and I immediately envision what my life will look like without the use of my right leg.

Paralyzed. Wheelchair bound. Dependent on my mother.

Dr. Anderson continues, "There is a chance that it will heal if the nerves regenerate, and overtime, parts of feeling may come back. When you become mobile, you will have to use a special device attached to your leg to help you walk, and you may need to use some sort of mobility aid for life. I don't have a crystal ball, so there's just no way of knowing for sure what the outcome will be. We will do testing in the future to measure the electrical activity of the nerves and muscles in your leg." He goes on to say that the only downside to the nerves healing would be the great pain and discomfort that I will have to endure.

Paralysis and *more pain? Wouldn't the upside of being paralyzed mean I can't feel* anything? The excitement and relief I have been living off of heading home begin slipping through my bruised fingers, along with my dreams of feeling the rush of adrenaline and dopamine that flood my body every time I run or work out. Moving my body is one of my greatest passions and one of the things that makes me who I am. *Is it going to be ripped away from me forever?* As Dr. Anderson continues explaining, I can hear a ringing in my ears and his voice just fades into the distance. I am genuinely trying to process what he is saying, but my mind won't let me go there.

"Your youth and determination are on your side." I snap back to the present to catch this detail. "Staying consistent with physical therapy is very important." And then he stops, takes a breath, puts his hand on my paralyzed leg and pats it reassuringly. "We will work together to find the best options for you as you continue to heal."

I take a deep breath, fighting like crazy to push away the feelings of panic and despair that are threatening to take me under.

I am only twenty-two years old. My life is just beginning and feels like it is over, all at once. It is a nightmare.

Dr. Anderson looks at me, a serious expression takes over his face and I notice his eyes are filled with concern. "Caitlin, do you understand what I am telling you?" he asks. I attempt to swallow the lump in my throat and draw in a deep breath, but I am hit with the harsh reality—I may never run again. Suppressing the urge to break down, especially in front of the surgeon who tirelessly fought to save my life, becomes my immediate priority. He's invested so much in me; I owe it to him to remain strong, to demonstrate that I can handle this setback.

"Yes, I understand," I manage to utter, my voice barely audible. Despite my efforts, tears threaten to overwhelm me, pooling in my eyes. But I staunchly refuse to let them spill. Succumbing to emotion would only make this grim reality too tangible.

Dr. Anderson's hand lands gently on my shoulder. "I'm sorry, Caitlin," his words seemed to mean more than sympathy. He had saved my life, but not my leg.

"Thank you for taking the time to explain things to me," I respond, pushing through the emotions that crack my voice. Sitting up a little straighter in my wheelchair, I look down at my right leg and make a split-second decision. "But I know that my leg will heal. I won't be using a mobility aid for the rest of my life."

"I truly hope and pray that is the outcome for you."

Dr. Anderson leans over to give me a hug, and I blurt out a muffled, "Thank you. I'll never be able to repay you for what you have done for me." Even amidst the heartache, I still have gratitude for being alive.

My mom turns to me and says, "I am so sorry about this news, Ca—"

"I am not going there," I interrupt, trying to push away the overwhelming emotions. "My leg will heal, Mom. This is not permanent," I snap, my frustration and fear taking over. I immediately regret my harsh tone with her. I take a deep breath and try to remain calm. My mind reels at the thought of my leg being paralyzed—*this kind of thing doesn't happen to a young girl like me. No, it must be a mistake. Surely, they've got it all wrong.*

Taking a deep, shuddering breath, I try to steady myself, to regain some semblance of composure amidst the chaos of my emotions. "I'm sorry, Mom. I just want to remain positive about this," I confess, my voice trembling with uncertainty and vulnerability.

"I get it. No more negative talk," she agrees.

The following morning, I wake up earlier than usual. My mom is bustling around, gathering our personal belongings. I can't imagine what I would want to keep from this experience, but she is filled with nervous energy, so it gives her something to do. I, too, am filled with a mixture of nerves and questions and wonderings; if only I could get up and move around to distract myself like she can.

Amidst the lingering anxiety of the news of my paralyzed leg, I still can't believe it. I am finally going home. It's been weeks of being cooped up in this sterile room. Finally, a change of scenery.

The ambulance would be arriving soon to transport both of us back the six hours it would take to get to my parents' house in Florida.

I am left alone as my mom continues her bustling, and my mind is still racing to process the news about my leg. I can't stop staring at it. Wrapped in a pink cast from hip to foot, all I can see are my toes poking out from the top. With all the determination I can muster, I gather my strength and will my toes to wiggle. *Come on, just move!!!!* I scream inside through gritted teeth. No movement. I try again, groaning with the effort, watching my toes closely, in case I miss even a fraction of movement. But there is no response. I let out my breath from all the effort and feel my heart sink even further.

If I could just get this cast off! I stick my fingers into the small space that is meant to support my nonmoving leg. It is hot and sweaty in there, and when I pull my fingers out, they smell rank. *Surely it's the weight of the cast that's keeping me from moving,* I convince myself. I cling to this thought desperately, denying the reality of my situation. I close my eyes as exhaustion creeps in and takes over, as it does most days.

"I hear you are anxious to go home. I'm John." A paramedic, ready to transport me home, wakes me from my short nap.

I attempt to smile, but the metal wires in my mouth remind me not to, of all the things to be self-conscious about, this is the worst part. A paramedic comes to each side of my hospital bed, and they carefully lift me onto the stretcher. My mom follows behind as they wheel me through the nurse-and-staff-lined hall. Encouraging words and farewells become a parade that I am the center of. Peggy, a nurse I had grown especially attached to, grabs my hand with a final plea, "Please come back and visit us one day. We are going to miss you!" Expressing my gratitude feels inadequate as I offer repeated thanks. "You've all been truly amazing. I'll never forget any of you," I assure them, my words imbued with genuine appreciation for their unwavering care and compassion.

As the two paramedics wheel me outside, I wonder if I am dreaming. Everything is in slow motion. The strong dose of morphine that had been given to me so I could tolerate the transport begins to take effect, and I can feel my eyelids growing heavy even though I desperately want to remember this moment, this freedom.

I can see the blurry figures of Dave and his mother, standing in front of me. Dave and his mother have been shuttling back and forth between their home in Austin and the hospital in Dallas. His mother's smile remains a source of comfort as she reaches for my hand, giving it a reassuring squeeze. "You focus on getting better, and let us know if you need anything, sweetie," she says. I nod, grateful for her kindness. Dave has plans to drive to Florida a few days after my arrival to help us settle into our new surroundings.

My mom climbs into the front seat of the ambulance and sandwiches herself between two paramedics: She's staring at her watch, mentally doing the math. It's 9:00 a.m., so we will be home by 6:00 p.m. I hear her trying to make small talk with them, but my mind is closing down in sleep.

I wake up a few hours later, curious to see where I am. The soft sound of country music greets me as I struggle to open my eyes. It takes me a moment to work out that I am no longer in my hospital room; a small bump swiftly reminds me I am not in my hospital bed anymore—I am homeward bound in an ambulance. Every movement, no matter how small, sends a sharp pain shooting up my spine. I wince and clench my teeth, wishing for the journey to be over.

I can hear my mom's voice coming from the front, chatting away with one of the paramedics about an episode of the *Oprah Winfrey Show*. I can't fully focus on their conversation, because my body is screaming for water. Even fully drugged, the parched feeling in my throat makes me feel like I might go crazy. "She's awake," Chris the paramedic, who has taken up his post next to me, announces to everyone in the ambulance. "How are you feeling?" I had been so out of it that I didn't even notice there was someone in the back of the ambulance with me.

"I need water," I rasp awkwardly. I try to open my mouth, but the wires make it difficult to form words. I watch desperately as he grabs a bottle of water and inserts a straw. He then kneels down on my level, allowing me to take a few sips. I close my eyes in relief. It tastes so good.

My mom hears me wrestling around and peers into the back of the ambulance to check on me. "Everything is just fine," Chris assures her.

I'm fine. I'm fine. I repeat this as my mantra even though each small bump and turn in the road sends waves of unrelenting pain through my body, causing my heart to race, and sweat to bead up on my upper lip. I know that if I don't get more medication soon, I will not be able to tolerate the remainder of the drive home.

"Are you feeling okay?" Chris asks, as he delicately places his fingers over my wrist to measure my pulse. I can't answer.

"I can tell you're in a lot of pain," he says, his concerned eyes meeting mine. Without hesitation, he springs into action, searching for the pain medications; it is only a matter of seconds before they are coursing through my system.

Forty minutes. That's how long it takes for pain medications to kick in. I take a few deep breaths and wait, trying to distract myself as I focus in on the inside of the ambulance and all the contraptions hanging from the ceiling. I suddenly realize I have a strong urge to urinate; my catheter, which was my normal mode of elimination, had been removed earlier, much to my relief. I was surprised to feel that I missed the convenience it offered.

I was in the most basic of predicaments. I had to wait for the pain medications to take effect before attempting to use the bathroom. There was no way I could handle even the slightest movement without them taking the edge off. Finally, after what feels like an eternity, the familiar numbing effects of the pain medications take over. I take a few moments to savor the relief of nothingness, but even still, my urge to empty my bladder is all I can think about.

"I need to get to a bathroom quickly," I say to Chris awkwardly through the wires in my mouth. He replies calmly that we will stop at the next gas station. *A gas station?* I immediately have images of the paramedics wheeling me in through a convenience store while I try not to wet myself. Before I can voice my concerns, the ambulance exits the highway and heads toward a gas station. John, the paramedic driving, flings the doors open and examines the parking lot. For what, I'm not sure. I feel the heaviness of my bladder threaten to give way and a cold wave of anxiety comes over me when he says, "This one won't work." He explains they are not able to carry me such a long distance and need to find a bathroom that is located on the exterior of the gas station. Unsure of how long I am capable of holding it, I nod in understanding. After the fourth attempt, the relief I feel when we *finally* find a gas station with an outdoor restroom facility is palpable. As John pulls the ambulance up as close as possible to the restroom, I can feel my nerves kicking in. I can see, from the stretcher I am strapped into, that my mom is understandably anxious about this transfer. She keeps asking the paramedics about the safety measures they will take. They quickly reassure her and promise they have it under control.

As John and Chris lift the stretcher out of the ambulance, I feel their gentle grip as they cradle me in their arms. Their hands tightly hook me underneath my armpits, ensuring that I am secure and comfortable. Mom darts off into the gas station to locate a key to the bathroom door. The next thing I know, I am being lifted onto the toilet by the paramedics. There is no time for modesty—if three's a crowd, then four is a show. As I prepare to let go, I am overcome by an excruciating pain near my tailbone, and I scream out in agony. My mom is right there, ready to take over with my toileting needs.

I desperately need to use the restroom, but the pain is unbearable, and my body just won't cooperate. It feels as if someone is stabbing me repeatedly in the tailbone. I sit there for several seconds, trying to relax through the pain and open up my bladder. I am wishing desperately for the toilet chair that had been so helpful to me in the hospital.

Finally, after what seems like an eternity, I am able to completely empty my bladder. This seemingly simple task is just another stark reminder of what I have been through. Even something as natural as peeing takes Herculean efforts thanks to the pelvic reconstructive surgery and nerve injuries.

As I am lifted off the toilet seat and transferred back into the ambulance, more pain medication is administered. *Will this ever end?* I wonder as I wait for the chemicals to erase the memory of what had just taken place. It's ironic. Before the accident, I had never taken more than an ibuprofen for the occasional headache. And here I am now, popping pain medication around the clock just so I can pee. I pass out again, even though I can still feel the familiar bumps and thuds of the ambulance against the pavement.

I am woken up abruptly by the delicious smell of frying food. The aroma of hamburgers and french fries hits my nostrils, and my eyes fly open. As if on cue, my stomach growls like it's got a wild animal inside it. It's lunchtime and John is making a pit stop for lunch at a roadside Krystal. I am so excited as I listen to him order for everyone in the ambulance. "I'd like a cheeseburger and french fries, please!" I blurt out my muffled order in between the wires in my mouth. I never really did care much for Krystal burgers, even though my dad frequently took my family there when I was a child, but after spending weeks slurping protein shakes and masticated food through a straw between the gap in my wires, I thought it sounded like the most glorious place on earth. Chris, with a look of confusion on his face, asked me to repeat myself. "I'd like a cheeseburger and french fries, please," I repeat as loud as I possibly can over the Krystal attendant's voice repeating their order over the loudspeaker. I'm as desperate for this burger as I was to pee. I watch amusement light up Chris's eyes as he tries to hold back a laugh. I know what he is thinking; there is no way I can eat a cheeseburger with my mouth wired shut. My mom, overhearing our conversation chimes in on Chris's behalf, "Cait, there's just no way you're going to be able to eat that."

"I can do it!" I was not going to let some measly wires stand between my stomach and this burger. I was done with pureed foods. I wanted some meat! Without hesitation, John puts in another order for a cheeseburger and fries. And with the help of my mom, who painstakingly mashes up tiny bits of cheeseburger and fries with her thumb and pointer finger, I am able to retrieve the small bits of burger and fries that she pushes through a small gap in my mouth with my tongue. It takes almost an hour, but I am able to consume half the burger and a small portion of fries. "It's like a mama bird feeding her baby bird," everyone jokes. To me, it was the best meal I had ever tasted. As we pass over the state line from Alabama to Florida, sleep takes over, and I slowly wake up from my drug-induced nap when the ambulance comes to a stop. I am dazed and confused, trying to make sense of my surroundings. The painkillers had knocked me out cold, but now I am wide awake. I wonder if we are home or if this is just another pit stop on our journey.

As if with some sort of grand ceremony, the paramedics open the doors of the ambulance . . . and I look out to be greeted by a dreary day. The sky is filled with dark, ominous clouds. But as my gaze shifts, I register familiar faces lining the driveway. Friends, family, and even my beloved dog are there to welcome me home.

Before I have time to process all the sensations going through my body and emotions moving through my heart, I am lifted out of the ambulance. I feel a comforting hand on my shoulder and know immediately it belongs to my grandfather. I look up to meet his eyes, both of us break down crying. Tears stream down my cheeks, staining my purple sweatshirt. My dad is by my side gently hugging me and then he lifts my dog up to my face. I sob even harder as I feel his wet tongue on my cheek, licking my tears away.

As they lift me into the wheelchair, I feel something crack open inside me. It's been held back for months—shock, grief, fear—all of it tumbling out in the silence between me and my dad as he grips the handles and pushes me forward. The driveway stretches out before us, the same driveway where I learned to ride a bike, where my rollerblades first met pavement. I can still picture the afternoons spent flying down it, legs strong, body light. Now, I sit here, weighed down by this chair, by the reality of how much has changed.

Ahead, the flowerbed comes into view. Azaleas, boxwoods, everything neatly trimmed and thriving. This used to be my jungle, where I hunted for lizards and frogs, collecting them in jars and letting my imagination run wild. But now, it looks like something from a different life. The wheelchair ramp leading to the front door is new, a gift from my uncle and dad, who spent weeks building it. Everyone tells me how thoughtful it is, but all I see is permanence—this glaring symbol of where I am and what I've lost.

My dad's hand lingers on my shoulder as we roll up the ramp. He doesn't say anything, but I don't need him to. The softness in his grip, the way his eyes dart toward me and then away—it all speaks louder than words. I know he's thinking about the daughter I used to be: fearless, always moving, always doing. And now here I am, stuck in this chair.

Inside the house, it's like stepping into a time capsule. Everything looks the same, but nothing feels right. Friends and family trail in behind me, their voices too loud, their faces too kind. I try to nod, to smile, to give them something that resembles normalcy, but I'm too tired. The ambulance ride drained me, and the pain hasn't left my body since the moment I woke up in the hospital. My uncle stands nearby, his face carved with concern. He doesn't say anything either, but his eyes betray him. They trace the sharp edges of my cheekbones, the hollows where muscle used to be, the way my arms and legs seem to shrink beneath me. I know what he sees because I see it too—a body that looks like it barely survived, a shadow of the person I once was.

I sit there, letting it all sink in. The weight of my dad's hand and the quiet sadness in the room. It's too much, but there's nowhere to escape. I can't run. I can't even stand. All I can do is sit here and try to hold it together, while every part of me feels like it's falling apart.

After an hour of visiting, the last guest finally exits our home. My mom wheels me to my room. Neither of us says a word. We are both exhausted. As we pass by the bathroom, I spot the shower bench and a newly installed handheld shower hose hanging off the tile wall. My dad had taken care of everything Dr. Anderson said I needed—while my mom had been attending to me in the hospital, he had put his fear and anxious energy into preparing, even the smallest details to make my life easier. My stomach lurched when I saw the toilet bench hovering over the stool, remembering the pain from our gas station stop earlier.

As my parents settle me into the comfort of my new hospital bed, my mom gently places the last dose of oxycodone into my hands. This, along with the fentanyl pain patches lining my back, offers some relief from the relentless pain that grips my body. With hopeful anticipation, I swallow the pills, hoping they will grant me the precious gift of sleep.

All I really want is a hot shower, to wash away the stress and pain of the day. But I know it is impossible right now. It's late, and the entire shower process would take nearly two hours. Even the simplest of tasks, such as changing my clothes, requires a great deal of effort. I reach for my glass of water and shake my head out of annoyance. The routine of taking medication has started to bother me greatly. It is a love-hate relationship. I know my survival depends on them, yet I wonder what the long-term implications will be. No one has mentioned that as a concern, and as I wonder if I'm the only one thinking about the lasting impact of these drugs, my mother's anxious voice breaks through my thoughts. "Cait, honey, will you be okay sleeping in here alone tonight?" This would be my first night without her, and I hesitate before responding with a half-hearted yes.

For the first time in my life, the prospect of being alone fills me with an unfamiliar dread. Once vibrant and full of life, I now harbor a profound distrust toward my own body, now a vessel of unpredictable agony capable of inflicting a torment so excruciating that it seems unbearable at times. It occurs to me that the car accident had shattered more than just bones; it had fractured my trust in my physical being. The image of waking up in that sterile hospital room, bound to the bed with mouth wired shut, flashes before my eyes with startling clarity. The sensation of choking on my own vomit, the bitter taste of fear lingering on my tongue, is a nightmare I can't shake. Memories press in on me from all sides, suffocating me with their weight. The fear of what my own my body is capable of, coupled with the lingering trauma of the near-death experience, leaves me feeling vulnerable and exposed in a way I have never felt before.

My mom leaves a cell phone by my bedside and instructs me to call her in the middle of the night if I need anything. As she moves toward the door, she takes one last look at me, as she turns out the lights. "Let me know if you need anything, Cait."

Panic starts to take over my mind and body, and I can feel my throat closing up. It chokes down any words of protest I might have been able to get out. I know my mom is exhausted, but my empathy for her is at war with my fear that I am going to die if I'm left here alone. It's been so long since I've slept by myself. What is going to happen to me if no one is right here, keeping watch? My panic turns to terror now that I am alone with the truth. There is no escaping this—my childhood bedroom was the place where my dreams were born, and now, I'm stuck in this nightmare, and my broken body won't let me leave. The gravity of my situation begins to set in. I had denied my way into believing, while I was in the hospital, that I had some sort of control over the outcome. But here, I can see clearly, in the dark—there is no cure, no remedy, no checklist that will speed up this process and offer me a way out. Utter hopelessness settles down into my lungs as I struggle to take a deep breath and move past my lack of control. I start to give in to the panic as tears stream down my face. Desperately seeking comfort, I clutch the pillow that was laid across my pelvis, as a protective barrier between me and the pain. I place it over my face and let out a close-mouthed scream, followed by uncontrollable sobs. I try to swallow them so that no one can hear me. I can't keep reality at bay any longer. For the first time since this nightmare began, I truly feel my mental state shift from hope to utter defeat. I pull the pillow down even harder over my face. I am slowly suffocating.

I eventually cry myself to sleep, but my escape from reality is short-lived, as I am torn from sleep by a fire-like pain engulfing the lower half of my body. My eyes roll back in my head as I try to breathe through it. Remembering I can call my mom, I reach for the cell phone and shakily dial her number. I don't want to wake her. I know she needs to rest, but I am desperate.

As I lay here in my bed, surrounded by the familiar walls of my childhood bedroom, I begrudgingly accept the truth. This was not the grand homecoming I had envisioned for myself. No. This is my new reality. I shift uncomfortably, the weight of my current situation pressing down on me like a leaden blanket.

I don't know if I have the strength to continue forward.

My room is silent, apart from the rhythmic ticking of the clock on the wall. The door creaks open. My mom enters bearing a plastic cup of painkillers.

"I know it's past time to take your pain medication," she murmurs, as she takes note of the look of agony etched on my face.

I nod wordlessly. Hands shaking, I reach for the white, circular tablets, swallowing them down with practiced ease.

I fix my gaze upon the clock, willing the hands to move faster. Just forty minutes until the searing torment subsides.

With a heavy heart, I close my eyes and cling to my pillow, grappling with the brutal truth of my circumstances before me. For the first time, I question God. *Why? What could possibly justify this pain?* I feel an intense sadness, anger, and shock all over again. As despair threatens to consume me whole, I realize there's no escaping this nightmare.

SEVEN

FIRE ANTS

Sweat drips down my face as I dart through the dense woods, my bare feet pounding the earth. My seven-year-old self is fueled by a fierce determination, a red flag tightly clutched in the back pocket of my Levi's denim shorts. I can hear the distant voices of my friends trailing behind me, urging me to slow down. Laughter bubbles up from the bottom of my belly. Speed is my superpower.

The shouts behind me grow fainter as I push myself deeper into the woods. A game of capture the flag is in full swing, and I have managed to steal the prized possession—the red flag. My heart races with excitement as I sprint toward our territory. Pausing for a brief moment to catch my breath, I quickly scan my surroundings, making sure no one is hiding nearby, waiting to snatch the flag from me. Satisfied that the coast is clear, I resume my sprint, determined to reach our fort and secure our victory.

Just as I am about to make my final dash, a searing pain shoots through both my feet. I know immediately what has happened—fire ants. Hundreds of them. Adrenaline courses through my body, temporarily numbing the pain, as I frantically brush the ants from the soles of my feet, crushing them in between my toes. Determined to secure a victory, I'm undeterred by my irritated and inflamed feet. I refuse to let that stop me.

Finally, I reach our fort and triumphantly place the red flag in an empty mason jar. "I win, I win, I win!" I declare myself the winner to anyone that can hear. My face is beaming with a wide grin, and I am too caught up in the moment to notice the pain inflicted by those venomous ants.

*   *   *

The moment I open my eyes, pain greets me. Like an unwelcome guest, it's simply too early to have to deal with something this severe. The sun is barely peeking through the blinds of my childhood bedroom, and I make out the shapes of my dresser, the chair in the corner piled with clothes, and my wheelchair. Unable to shift my body from side to side, I recline my hospital bed into an upright position, a desperate attempt to find relief from pain that courses through me. I feel as though my body has been stuffed in a cardboard box, and I have been unable to shift or rotate my position for days on end. It's the consequences of shattered bones and severe nerve damage.

As I lie there, I reflect again on my encounter with the fire ants. But this time, it's not just a memory—it's a reality. My body is wracked with pain. The fire-like sensation radiates from the bottom of my feet up through my broken body, weaving its way through my shattered pelvis, settling in my tailbone. It's as if I am being eaten alive by vicious, red-colored ants, only this time it is from the inside out. As a child, it felt like the worst pain I had ever experienced, but even as a child, I was confident that it would eventually subside. This pain is unrelenting, all consuming. It never leaves, not even in my dreams.

My thoughts are interrupted by a knock at my bedroom door and my in-home healthcare nurse enters my room before I can answer. She's new and I stare at her blankly as she introduces herself. "Hi, Caitlin, I'm Shannon. I'll be your nurse for the next couple of months."

I have mixed feelings about Shannon. On one hand, I am happy to see a new face, but on the other, my injuries have left me feeling guarded and protective over my fragile body, and I wondered if she is up to speed on my medical history.

Shannon helps me sit up and scoots me to the edge of the bed. "Let's get you changed into something other than your pajamas before I take your vitals, and then we can chat about your medical history. What would you like to wear today?" She asks. At this point, I was rotating between an oversized pair of black and gray sweatpants, and several loose-fitting T-shirts I had accumulated over the years. I motion toward the black pants folded on my dresser. "My T-shirts are in my top drawer. Just surprise me," I answer, grateful for her assistance.

I feel relieved to no longer be wearing a hospital gown. Regular clothes offer a semblance of normalcy. Even if it's shapeless sweatpants and ratty old T-shirts from high school. I'm grateful to have a new collection of soft nightgowns thanks to a thoughtful gesture from my mom's friend, streamlining the undressing and dressing process, alleviating the hassle of struggling to get pajama pants over a leg cast. Shannon helps me as I carefully remove the turquoise gown over my head. I groan in agony. Even the small motion of lifting my arms up into the air causes pain to rip through my pelvic region. I have to move at a slower pace.

The next part is tricky. Before the accident, I could never have imagined what a daunting task putting on a pair of pants could be. Shannon gently assists me and together, we navigate the pants over my pink cast, rolling them inch by inch toward my pelvis. As she progresses closer to my pelvic area, I instinctively put my hand out to halt her movement. She stops abruptly and backs away a few inches. "Is everything alright?" I hesitate and snap my hand back onto the bed. I nervously admit that I'm in so much pain all the time that I worry about even the slightest touch adding to my torture. She nods sympathetically and assures me she will take great care. I almost sag with relief. At last, I'm dressed. *With no place to go!* I pull myself upright in my hospital bed, and reach for my handheld mirror on the nightstand, intending to tackle the tangled mess of yesterday's hair tie. I sigh heavily as I survey my hair, a greasy mess of tangled strands.

It's just another reminder of my inability to maintain my usual hygiene standards. Before, I was meticulous about cleanliness, so being unable to attend to my personal grooming needs such as showering regularly and washing my hair, is incredibly frustrating. As Shannon sifts through my paperwork, I hastily pull my hair into a bun that sits lopsided on the top of my head. I realize I've forgotten to apply deodorant prior to dressing, and feel annoyed that I'm going to have to ask Shannon to fetch it for me. I'm at the end of my rope when it comes to asking people to help me. Independence has always been my strong suit, and I notice myself shifting to an older mindset, worried I'm going to come across as demanding. It takes as much strength to remind myself that Shannon is here for the purpose of helping me. I push past my pride and frustration as I scold myself. *Get a grip, Caitlin. Just ask her to find your deodorant.*

Shannon looks up from her paperwork and her eyes meet mine.

"Do you need me to get you something?" She intuitively surmises.

"I can't seem to find my deodorant,"

"Oh! I guess we missed that step," she laughs. Shannon retrieves my deodorant from the drawer inside my nightstand, where my mom had placed a handful of toiletry items for easy access.

Now that my deodorant is applied and hair is in place, I feel ready to tackle the next task: delving into my medical history.

"My surgeon compared me to a frog thrown in a blender," I casually blurt out, recalling the conversation where my surgeon stressed the importance of sharing my medical backstory with anyone attending to my care. Shannon's eyes widened at my unexpected analogy.

"Wow," she responds, clearly taken aback. "As I'm going through your medical history, it's evident that your insides went through significant trauma."

I mentally acknowledge her comprehension of the situation.

"It's incredible to think that none of your internal organs were pierced by the bone fragments," she added.

"Yeah, my surgeon told my folks it was a miracle that my organs came out unscathed. He kept saying it was as if my bones broke in strategic positions all around my organs."

Shannon continues to express her astonishment, repeatedly murmuring "wow" as she examines my X-rays.

Okay. She gets it, I think to myself, now embarrassed about my hesitation to ask her about the deodorant.

We chat a bit longer as she takes my vitals. Everything checks out good. My blood pressure is normal. For now, anyway. It always seems to spike when my pain levels are out of control, I explain to her. She gives me a plastic cup with a handful of medications. "Oh, you're on fentanyl," she remarks with surprise. "I'm not accustomed to working with patients who are prescribed a potent medication like fentanyl. Is someone monitoring this for you? I know it can be very dangerous if not administered properly." She looks at me with discomfort as she brings the water bottle over to me.

I suppose she's not familiar with handling trauma cases after all.

"My mom was schooled during my hospital stay on how to properly administer the patch, and I know she is staying in close communication with my surgeon and his nurse," I explain, trying to communicate to her that we have it under control.

"That makes me feel better," Shannon replies, a look of relief crossing her face.

She flips through my paperwork once more and exclaims, "Oh, we missed something!" I immediately know what she's referring to. Another day, another jab in the stomach. "How could we forget?" I tease. Shannon pulls up my shirt and inspects my bruised abdomen.

"Wow, you're really black and blue," she remarks. I roll my eyes inwardly, just wanting to get it over with—I don't need these useless observations. I close my eyes, avoiding the sight of my battle scars. I've lost count of the many times I've been poked by needles in the stomach, arms, and legs.

Shannon administers the Fragmin shot before asking, "Is there anything else you need from me before I go? A bathroom break?"

I suddenly realize I've been holding my bladder ever since Shannon arrived. "Actually, I really need to use the restroom," I admit. Without hesitation, Shannon assists me into my wheelchair and wheels me to the bathroom. After taking care of business, Shannon guides me back to my bed and hands me two oxycodone tablets. I gulp them down right away through a small opening between my teeth. My stomach rumbles, reminding me that I haven't eaten anything all morning.

"See you bright and early tomorrow," Shannon smiles on her way out of the room. As the familiar warmth of my pain medication begins to slowly course through my body, my mom appears with a steaming bowl of my all-time favorite comfort food: chicken and dumplings. With a soft plastic baby spoon in hand, she carefully places the bowl on the wicker tray that my papa had thoughtfully lent me. I feel a sense of nostalgia as I gaze at the familiar dish, positioned on a pillow over my midsection.

I am immediately transported back to my childhood when I would spend time at my great-grandmother's house. I can still remember standing on a step stool in her kitchen, eagerly helping her roll out the dumplings. And when she wasn't looking, or so I thought, I would sneak a few bites, relishing in the deliciousness. She would point her finger at me and declare, "That's my feisty one."

Taking my first bite of the steaming dish, my mouth fills with the familiar taste and texture of her dumplings—and my heart fills with fondness at the comforting memory of her.

I take small, painstakingly safe bites, maneuvering around and through my wired mouth, thinking about how word has quickly spread in our small town about my particular love for chicken and dumplings. As a result, several pots of the dish have magically appeared on our doorstep. So many pots, in fact, that my mom has resorted to freezing them to make room in the fridge.

It may have taken me nearly twenty minutes to finish the small bowl, but it was worth every slow and deliberate bite. My stomach gurgles in agreement. I would go on to eat chicken and dumplings for breakfast, lunch, and dinner on my hard days, much to the amusement of my family.

The hours drag on at an excruciatingly slow pace. Each hour of agony and boredom I endure in my hospital bed gets me closer to my next dose of painkillers. I swallow my third dose, praying it numbs both my body and mind. Sleep claims me for an hour and relief is fleeting. I'm still in that space where sleep and awake collide when the creak of the front door echoes through the house. I tense up when I hear the familiar voice.

It's Dave.

My mom mentioned his potential arrival sometime this week. *Why didn't he bother with a courtesy call—or at the very least—a text beforehand?*

He has traveled from Austin to spend two weeks with my family in Florida, and maintains it is to help us adjust to our new lifestyle. My sister slips into my room, sealing us off from Dave and the outside world with the click of the door. "Dave's here," she announces hesitantly, as if I hadn't already heard his arrival. "I know," I reply flatly, my voice betraying my lack of enthusiasm.

She sees right through my façade and continues, "He says he came to help with the adjustment and is planning on staying here for two weeks. . . . What do you think about that?" She gives me no time to reply before she answers for me, "I don't know if I can handle being around him for that long."

"I don't know what to think," I snap. "I am just taking it one day at a time." She studies me for a moment and answers, "Well, you know you can tell him to leave if you're not comfortable with him being here."

"He's still my boyfriend, Ash," I remind her with exasperation.

"I'm well aware," she replies, rolling her eyes as she turns the knob, pulls open the door. She gives me a look that says it all: *Why would I want to stay with the guy whose reckless ways nearly killed me?*

Once again, I'm left alone with my thoughts. And they are all over the place.

Just breathe. I remind myself. Without the haze of morphine to cloud my senses, I'm acutely aware of the weight of unanswered questions pressing down on me. But the memory of Dave's anger, as well as his impatience, keeps me from broaching the subject of the accident again. *I'll wait*, I decide. *But how long will I keep avoiding the inevitable? I know there is more to the story. The accident. The deer. I have so many lingering questions.*

My thoughts are interrupted by the sound of footsteps approaching my room. My palms begin to sweat, and I push my hands further underneath the sheets. *Why am I so nervous?* I had seen Dave hundreds of times before. But this time feels different. He is on my turf now. I recall my dad's expression when I told him Dave would be staying with us for two weeks. The deep inhale and clenched jaw said everything—he was far from pleased.

As my mind wanders, the creak of my bedroom door brings it back to the present. There stands Dave, a bouquet of vibrant red roses obscuring his face. I shoot a disdainful glance at the flowers.

Roses won't fix me, I muse, watching as Dave places them on my dresser.

"I saw these and thought they might brighten your day," he says, taking a seat on the edge of my bed. I struggle to spit out even a simple thank you, my expression blank as I stare at the wall in front of me. I feel his eyes on me, sizing me up, like a hawk would its prey.

"You look like hell," he blurts out. I remain silent, refusing to look at him, but inside, I am seething.

No kidding. Bitter retorts bubble up in my throat, but I shove them back down. Sensing my frustration, Dave attempts to backtrack. "You just don't look like yourself anymore," he stammers, digging himself deeper into a hole created by his own stupidity.

"Thanks for the insight," I snap, moving my hands back on top of the sheet. Dave tries to speak again, but I promptly cut him off before he can even start. "Can you just . . . stop?" My body trembles, pulsing with pain, but I push through, driven to make my point.

"Listen, I know appearances matter to you, but right now, my physical state is the least of my concerns!"

Dave goes silent.

I motion down at my once-toned legs now wasted, covered by a cast and old sweat pants; I am aware of the toll the injuries have taken on my body. I had only seen myself from the neck up using a small, handheld mirror, where I took note of my hollow cheeks, dark under-eye circles, and pale complexion.

I can practically feel Dave's disappointment radiating off him as my voice raises higher; I'm broken and bruised, no longer fit to be his decorative accessory. And I'm mad.

"You're the most self-absorbed asshole I've ever met!" I scream right into his face. He blinks once, then twice and says simply, "Wow." He is stunned by my reaction.

Taking a deep breath and dismissing my feelings, Dave prattles on about something he did last week. I tune him out, fixating on the roses. I imagine hurling the entire vase against the wall and the satisfaction I would feel as I watched them crumble into a hundred pieces.

"Are you even listening?" Dave snaps his fingers in front of my face, jolting me back to reality. "Yes," I reply, my voice tight, though his words barely register.

We are both surprised as my bedroom door swings open. "Everything okay in here?" my sister asks, carefully observing my eyes.

"We are just fine," I respond sharply.

"Just checking!" she croons, shooting Dave a hateful glance as she closes the door behind her. I take a few moments to breathe and calm myself down.

Dave rummages through his backpack producing a brand-new video camera. "While I visit, my dad thought we should document your progress," he explains casually. Unbeknownst to me, his father had been whispering about lawsuits and insurance claims to my dad from behind closed doors. My dad was waiting for the right time to drop this bombshell on me.

"Umm . . . I guess . . ." I feel even more confused and exhausted. Pleased with my compliance, Dave gets to work setting up the camera. I take a few minutes to rest my eyes. "I'm off to grab lunch. Starving," Dave announces, leaving the camera on my dresser.

"Need me to grab you anything?" he offers as he pulls the door open. "Nah," I reply, clutching the pillow on my lap a little tighter.

Dave is nowhere to be found for the remainder of the day. It turns out that he stumbled upon someone selling a new AR rifle just thirty minutes south of us, so he took off to snag it after he grabbed lunch. Characterized by his fervent enthusiasm for firearms and a propensity for extravagant spending, his impulsivity comes as no surprise. No surprise he spun a cover story with ease, telling his father the money had gone toward buying medical supplies for me. I sat in stunned silence listening as the lie rolled effortlessly off his tongue—like it was second nature.

I remain confined to my hospital bed for the better part of the day, except for a few short trips around the house being pushed in my wheelchair. I am grateful for the reclining feature on the wheelchair which provides crucial support for my body, as well as the elevated leg rest. However, even with these accommodations, my ability to maintain even a slightly upright position is severely limited. I have worked my way up to almost fifteen minutes in the wheelchair before the pain from the pressure on my tailbone becomes overwhelming and intolerable.

As evening approaches, Dave has returned and my pain levels become increasingly worse—it comes in relentless waves that seem to seep into every corner of my body. My mom brings me dinner, but I refuse to eat. I can hardly see straight from the pain.

As it escalates, the lower half of my body feels like acid is coursing through my veins. I tightly grip the sides of my bed sheets while my sister soothes me, gently rubbing my head, while I moan in agony. Dave has disappeared, holed up in the far bedroom, engrossed in his Xbox, oblivious to my distress.

"It's getting worse, it feels like I'm on fire!" I scream and cry. "I can't take it anymore; I just can't! Get me back to the hospital! I need to get out of here!" Panic overwhelms me as I beg God, my sister, anyone listening, for some relief.

My mom stands by my dad, tears welling up in her eyes, while he frantically tries to reach my surgeon in Dallas. "We are on hold," my dad whispers helplessly. Electric shocks of pain jolt through me relentlessly, from my tailbone down to my feet, each surge more excruciating than the last. I lie there, trapped on my back, my nightgown plastered to my sweat-drenched skin, afraid to so much as twitch for fear of unleashing an even greater torment.

Another wave of pain rips down the sides of my legs, shooting out through my big toes like bolts of lightning. With each pulse of pain, I feel like I'm being torn apart from the inside out. In a frenzy of anguish, I claw at my own scalp, ripping out clumps of my hair.

"God, please," I gasp the words out as a raw plea; I beg for a reprieve that seems hopelessly out of reach.

"Cait, please stop!" My sister is crying as she tries to keep my hands away from my scalp. "This is crazy. Can't we just take her to the ER?" My dad steps out of the room, struggling to hear the doctor over my piercing screams.

"Her pain is off the charts, and she's tearing her hair out!" My dad is practically shouting, desperately trying to urgently convey the gravity of the situation.

Dr. Anderson is put on the phone and remains calm as he attempts to reassure my dad. "We are going to do everything we can to help her. Can you describe the type of pain she's feeling?"

"It's like an intense burning that is shooting down from her tailbone," my dad explains.

"It sounds like the nerves are starting to wake up and fire," Dr. Anderson responds with confidence, as if he anticipated this outcome. "This is actually a positive sign as it indicates nerve regeneration, but unfortunately, it also can mean excruciating pain for the patient. Given that her sciatic nerve was severed, along with severe damage to the surrounding nerves in her pelvis, sudden increases in pain are likely."

My dad maintains a steady nod as he replies, "Yeah, alright. I understand."

"We need to up her dosage of Lyrica right away," Dr. Anderson instructs, referring to my nerve-pain medication.

"Got it," my dad acknowledges. "I have a friend who's a pharmacist. I'll call him as soon as I hang up and see if he can get it to us tonight. She really can't endure this without it."

Dr. Anderson emphasizes the importance of watching my blood pressure and gives the go ahead to take me to the ER if the additional meds don't provide relief. In the midst of my ongoing screams and tears, it dawns on me why Dr. Anderson inquired about my home life at the rehab hospital. He knew the challenges

I would soon be up against and wanted to be sure I was returning to an environment that could meet the challenges. It also becomes clear why he was hesitant about my early discharge from the hospital.

I am so stupid. I shouldn't have rushed to get out of there. I sob into my hands as I try to breathe through the pain.

"What's happening?" Dave has heard the screaming.

"Cait's pain is out of control!" my sister shouts at him in accusation.

With a look of astonishment plastered across his face, Dave hurriedly approaches my bed, pushing my sister aside as he places a hand on my shoulder. "Why isn't anyone taking action?" he asks with evident frustration. "Where are more pain meds?!"

Not in the mood to be ordered around, my mom steps in and explains that the dose I have been given is not alleviating the nerve pain. "Oxycodone and fentanyl won't provide relief for this type of pain. Her dad is currently on the phone trying to get another medication filled at the pharmacy."

Dad manages to reach his friend Dave, our trusted local pharmacist, and quickly fills him in on the situation. Without a moment's hesitation, Dave prepares the medication and instructs my dad to come pick it up.

By this point, my legs and feet have become so hypersensitive that even the gentle touch of a light sheet on my toes feels unbearable. It is akin to having my legs ensnared in live wires that are constantly sparking and firing. As adrenaline surges through my body, my heart rate soars, consequently elevating my blood pressure.

Mom retrieves the blood pressure device left behind by the in-home healthcare nurse to monitor it. The reading displayed 170/95.

Hurry up, Dad!

After what feels like an eternity, my dad bursts through my bedroom door, medication in hand. He's shaking as he passes me the pills, and I practically choke on the water as I desperately swallow them down.

I try to ease into relaxation, but my body won't allow it. All control is lost, having slipped through my fingers like sand. My legs are a sickly hue of purple, toes contorted and curling inward. I feel like I am on fire while an invisible force crushes my bones in my legs and pelvis. The agony consumes me, pushing me to the brink of insanity. In this moment, with everyone standing around me, I want to die. Dying would mean freedom from this relentless torment.

I'm suddenly hit with the urgent need to use the bathroom. The nerve damage around my pelvis has robbed me of bladder control. "I'm going to wet myself!" I scream desperately, unable to move. With Mom's careful assistance, I settle into my wheelchair, clinging to one last shred of dignity as we head toward the bathroom. As I'm lifted out of the wheelchair and reach for the walker placed in front of the toilet, I feel the warm trickle of urine streaming down my legs, and watch helplessly as a puddle of pee forms on the floor. The sharp scent of urine fills the air and I'm engulfed in a wave of defeat, consumed by self-pity and shame. My mom and I lock eyes, and a flood of tears erupt from both of us as she pulls my broken body into a hug. Our shared frustration and exhaustion spill onto the floor, mixing with the puddle of urine. I ache as I register the exhaustion on my mother's face as she gently wipes the urine from my legs with a damp cloth. Too tired to speak, she silently dresses me in a fresh nightgown before helping me back into my hospital bed. After about an hour, the intense burning starts to ease up a bit. Despite the persistent discomfort and unrelenting pain, I experience a glimmer of relief—the medication has begun to take the edge off my suffering.

I ask my mom to bring me a double dose of oxycodone, desperately hoping it will finally grant me some peace in the form of sleep. I instinctively pop the painkillers into my mouth, it's become second nature to me. Exhaustion weighs heavily on my parents, and they slip off to bed, seeking their own solace. With a tired sigh, my sister quietly slips out my bedroom door.

Emotionally and physically drained, I unravel once more, tears flowing freely down my cheeks and pooling into the sides of my greasy hair. Dave makes his way to the door, pauses, and before leaving turns back to me and says simply, "Just go to sleep and quit feeling sorry for yourself. You'll feel better in the morning." Choking back sobs I wonder, *Did I hear him correctly?* Lacking the energy to muster any response or defense I lay silent in my hospital bed, defeated. I simply sink deeper into my covers, longing for the oblivion of medicated sleep to take over.

My sister, lingering by the door of her bedroom, overheard Dave. She was as baffled as I was. Later, she would confide in me, with eyes blazing, that it took all her strength not to cross the hall and punch Dave square in the face. *How could he say such things?* she would wonder aloud. The audacity of his words left her fuming inside. However, rather than acting on her impulse, she pulled out her journal as a means to process the events of the night.

Lying there, my body motionless, I drift back to memories of being that carefree seven-year-old, racing barefoot through the woods. She had no clue what lay ahead—the battles she'd face, the pain that would grip her.

Will I ever feel that innocent joy again? I ponder. *Will I be able to push through the trials before me and emerge victoriously like I did when I proudly seized that crimson flag?* Oh, how I longed to return to that girl, running wild and free through the untamed forest with reckless abandon, the only thing burning her being those pesky fire ants.

EIGHT

BOMBSHELL

For days, I plead with anyone within earshot to take me back to the hospital. "Even if it means navigating my wheelchair solo all the way back to Dallas, I'm going!" I declare, fueled by the torture my pain is causing. The frustration consumes me, leaving me breathless and sweating in my hospital bed, fighting despair and defeat.

My mom thinks a change of scenery might help the darkness taking over, and so she wheels me over to the open back door, encouraging me to take deep drags of fresh air into my body. Dave has hardly left the guest room, and when he does, he is immersed in his own world made possible by headphones that are glued to his ears. He takes refuge in his Xbox, and once again, leaves me stranded, fighting for my life. As I suck down the tail end of the breeze that drifts by, I envision being back at the rehab hospital, my craving for the numbing effects of the morphine have overtaken my yearning to be home, in my own bed. No matter how hard I beg, I cannot escape this overwhelming reality.

Why did I want to leave so soon? I wrestle with this question endlessly, grappling with the silence of God. Despite my mom's attempts to console me with scripture during my hospital stay, the words ring hollow. *How can anything good possibly emerge from this ordeal?*

Dave pauses his Xbox session, pulls his headphones off as he glances over at me. "Feel like some fresh air?"

I hesitate before responding. Anger still courses through me, fueled by the hurtful comment he made the other night. The audacity of implying I'm just feeling sorry for myself—I can't let it go. It still stings.

And then it finally dawns on me—his lack of understanding. He can't possibly comprehend the depths of my pain. Memories flash through my mind that give me the proof I need to come to this understanding. Like when he clumsily fell from a moped suffering only a minor scrape. He handled it like a child toppling from a bike, shouting and clawing at the pavement, his body trembling uncontrollably.

Despite my lingering resentment, the allure of escaping the confines of this house is undeniable. As someone who loves sunshine and being outdoors, the walls are suffocating. Reluctantly, I acquiesce.

"Yes, but I can't promise I'll last long sitting upright," I admit.

"We'll make it quick," he assures, guiding me toward the front door and once through it, down the ramp.

As I'm wheeled into the sunlight, I'm immediately greeted by its comforting warmth, a sensation I haven't felt in what feels like an eternity. I glance up at the deep, blue sky—it's as if the world has never looked quite so magnificent. Perhaps I was just too busy to appreciate the beauty that surrounded me prior to my accident.

Dave slowly pushes me down the driveway and back. With my eyes closed, I bask in the sun's warmth, wishing time would stand still and that my body would cooperate. Surprisingly, the pain that continues to plague me eases up a bit, as if the sunshine is working its magic on me.

"Ready to call it quits?" Dave asks.

"Not just yet," I murmur, relishing every second of this rare moment of serenity. Inwardly, I offer a silent prayer of gratitude for the sun's warmth. I can't believe it. I have managed to stay in my wheelchair for a full twenty minutes, a new personal record.

Progress, I whisper to myself.

Dave gently maneuvers my wheelchair back indoors, and as the sun turns to shadow, I can't ignore the discomfort creeping in from where the sun left off. My legs feel oddly contorted due to the nerve damage, and a dull ache radiates downward from my tailbone. Despite my reluctance to let go of the blissful moment outside, I realize the urgency of returning to my hospital bed before the pain worsens. With Dave's assistance, I transition back to my hospital bed, sinking into its familiarity. Though I still crave the sun's warmth, there is a feeling of relief when I am able to recline back into bed.

"Dave, we need to talk about the night of the accident," I blurt out. I hadn't been ready to talk about it in the immediate aftermath of my own survival but bolstered by the sun and my own recognition of progress, I know it is time.

"Oh, here we go again," Dave grumbles to no one in particular.

"Yes, this again." My patience is wearing thin. "I need answers! It's not right that I can't remember anything from that night, and I'm left to worry over what really happened." My voice grows more intense with each word. *I want answers. And I want them now.*

"I guess you just don't trust me, huh?" Dave challenges me with a look that says he will do whatever he has to do to protect himself. I get a shiver that lodges in my throbbing back.

"No, I don't," I reply firmly. "Call it women's intuition if you will, but I've never bought into the excuse that a deer caused the accident. You were going way too fast. I remember that. There's no way you could have spotted a deer and reacted in time to swerve. It just doesn't add." As I mull over the myriad of possibilities, one thing remains clear: Dave's penchant for high-speed driving, well beyond the limits of reason, had something to do with why my body is fractured and I am confined to this bed. Memories flood back of many tumultuous rides together—me clinging to the door handle, white-knuckled, begging him to ease off the throttle.

Often, my pleas were met with a barrage of curses or dismissive commands occasionally punctuated by a ripple of unsettling laughter, as though my panic amused him.

I also can't discount the possibility of substance abuse. Dave had mentioned to me a while back that his close friend was dabbling in hardcore drugs, particularly during weekend binges, adding another layer of uncertainty to an already murky situation. I had never personally witnessed Dave using drugs, but that didn't mean he hadn't. I found it interesting, and perhaps pertinent, that Dave had admitted to spending a few hours at this friend's house in Austin prior to picking me up from the airport the night of the accident.

Watching him cautiously, I decide to switch gears. Instead of drilling him with questions, I lay out potential scenarios. I take up the role of a cross-examining detective—like the ones I watch in my beloved true crime docuseries. I want to paint a picture of that night and see what sticks.

I take a deep breath and reposition my body to ease the pressure on my pelvis. *Here goes nothing.*

"Maybe you stopped by Daniel's place and had a bit too much to drink—or tried something else that impaired your senses. Then, you came to pick me up from the airport, thinking you'd gotten away with it. But whatever you had taken was still in your system, clouding your judgment. Maybe you thought you saw something—a deer, perhaps. But you were driving too fast, and before you knew it, you lost control of the car. And that's how we ended up in that accident."

There, I said it. With each word, I watch for his reaction, hoping to catch a glimpse of truth amidst the tangled web of possibilities.

Dave's face flushes red, the veins in his forehead pulsate as he attempts to restrain himself from lashing out at me. Yet, he remains silent, his gaze fixed on the floor.

Very un-Dave-like, I think to myself.

I quickly realize that the presence of my family in my home is likely what's preventing him from letting his anger loose. And I take my opportunity, because I know I'm safe.

"Well?" I prompt, eager for his response.

To my astonishment, Dave bursts into laughter. His tone drips with sarcasm as he mocks my attempts to unravel his secrets. His nervous energy is that of a child, caught—and there is no turning back.

"I'm confused!" I admit, struggling to comprehend his reaction.

"Congratulations, Sherlock, you have finally cracked the case—there was no deer," he reveals with a mocking sneer, as he claps his hands in front of my face.

His words strike me like a blow to the chest. The air escapes my lungs in a rush as I struggle to process his admission.

"What?" I manage to gasp, my voice trembling with disbelief at his response, utterly stunned by what I've just heard.

"I had a few drinks and took some pills at Daniel's, but so what? That was hours before I picked you up from the airport. It

didn't impair my judgment." His tone, so matter of fact, is mysti-
fying.

"I was just speeding in the rain, lost control like an idiot, and
panicked. That's why I made up a bullshit story about the deer. But
keep your mouth shut. I could get screwed over big time," he warns
me bluntly, his gaze holds me down onto my bed. Even if I could
get myself up, I wouldn't be able to.

I'm at a loss for words and cover my face with trembling
hands; so many feelings build up inside me and I'm afraid of what
is coming next. "They tested me for drugs at the hospital," he
proceeds boldly. "I haven't heard anything, so I assume I'm in the
clear."

"Since when did you start taking pills?" I demand, confused,
frustrated, fragmented. I shake my head as if to free my thinking
from everything he has just revealed. I can't make sense of it and
all I can do is scream. "Just LEAVE!" I explode, unable to bear his
presence any longer—I need him to go, *now*.

Dave chuckles nervously, attempting to downplay the severity of the situation. "You don't really want me to leave. It's not a big
deal. I did what I thought was best for both of us."

"For both of us or just for yourself?" My voice is at a decibel
so loud, I didn't know I could make that much noise. "Just go!" I
shout, my patience for him and the mess he has created has evap-
orated.

Dave rises from the bed, his movement hesitant. He lingers
at the door, turning back to glare at me. "Not a word of this to
anyone," he warns.

My sister must have heard the commotion in the next room over. I hear her talking to Dave out in the hall. "She hates me," he whines to her.

Always the victim. My body shakes as it begins to absorb the truth.

"Well, I'm not surprised," she is looking right at me as she walks into my room, shutting the door behind her. My brain is in overdrive as I scramble to wrap my head around the bombshell that just exploded in my face.

Why am I so surprised? Dave's a master at dancing around the truth. *Do I tell someone?* I have to tell someone.

"What's going on, Cait?" my sister asks, taking note of my distress and Dave's stomping and door slamming at the other end of the hall. "I just need some time alone to think things through. We can talk about it later." I'm not ready to process this with anyone else yet.

As night approaches, I am too overwhelmed with grief to sleep. I feel betrayed. How many more lies has he told to save himself? My mom and dad pop in to check on me before going to bed. One look tells them everything they need to know; something isn't right. "Dave and I had a fight, and I told him to leave," I blurt out.

Even in my emotional and physical pain, I don't miss the flicker of relief in my dad's eyes.

"I'm sorry," my mom says quietly. "Is there anything we can do for you?" her voice is filled with genuine concern.

"Nah, just need my pain meds to help me sleep," I respond, hoping to cut the conversation short.

"Before we turn in, there's something I need to talk to you about," my dad confesses.

I note his serious tone immediately—my heart sinks. I can't handle any more hard truths right now.

"Dave's dad approached me when I was at the hospital visiting you," my dad continues. "He was flipping through your medical records while the doctor was busy, and then he pulled me aside. He wants you to sue him. He says the insurance company will be responsible for paying out."

"Sue him?" I blurt out, my voice trembling in disbelief.

"It's just something to consider, we don't know what the future holds for you, Cait."

"No, absolutely not," I interject firmly. "And I don't want to hear about it again."

My dad turns to leave the room, but before he exits says, "Just think about it, Cait. That's all I'm asking. I'm genuinely concerned about your future."

Why is everyone so worried about my future? I huff and cross my arms over my chest. I need this day to be over.

My mom, still sitting at the edge of my bed, gently massages my throbbing head. "I can't believe this is my life," I sob, tears streaming down my cheeks. "I should be gearing up for my senior trip, ready to hike the Grand Canyon from rim to rim with Dawna.

Instead, I'm stuck in this bed, broken, and in pain. It feels like my life is over, Mom."

"Don't say that, Cait," she whispers, gently pulling strands of hair away from my tear-stained face and tucking them behind my ear. "You never know what God has in store for you."

"Yeah, I've heard that line before, along with the classic 'God won't give you more than you can handle,'" I reply bitterly. "But life isn't all sunshine and rainbows. People go through tough stuff, you know?"

"I know, Cait," my mom sighs. "You've faced more challenges in the past few months than most people do in a lifetime. You are so strong. Don't lose hope. Remember the verse I shared with you in the hospital? Romans 8:28—'We know that all things work together for good.' I truly believe that something good will come from all this pain."

I bury my face in my pillow, unable to find the words to respond.

"Try to get some sleep, Cait. And I'm a phone call away if you need anything. The cell phone is next to your bed."

Mom quietly leaves my room and shuts off the light.

I snatch the pillow away from my face, and a wave of anger hits me with the force of a tsunami. It wells up inside me and I feel like I'm going to drown. Choking on the emotion, all aimed at Dave, I find somewhere, mixed in with all my fury that I have some to spare for God and this whole messed up situation. My fists clench around the pillow, a primal urge to sink my teeth into it comes over me. I'm even more incensed when I can't because my mouth remains sealed by wires. Every fiber of my being yearns to thrash and twist in bed, to release the pent-up frustration that has lodged in my broken bones, but I can't. I'm confined to lying flat on my back. I crave the freedom to lace up my sneakers and pound the pavement, to run until I can no longer feel the ache in my bones and the despair in my heart. The days of waking up feeling energized and ready to tackle the day are now just a distant memory. Instead, fatigue, pain, and chronic dehydration are all that meet me. The relentless struggle against extreme constipation adds another layer of discomfort to my already burdened body.

I'm jolted awake—*How had I fallen asleep while I was so furious and distraught last night?!*—when I feel the familiar pain in my stomach caused by severe constipation. It is similar to how it felt at the rehab hospital, and I need an enema—fast. I reach for the cell phone and call my parents' house phone. My mom doesn't answer but instead bolts through my bedroom door.

"Everything okay?"

"I'm in serious pain and I need water, Mom."

"Okay, just a minute." She leaves the room and is back in a flash.

"Here take these," she says, handing me the all too familiar painkillers. I drink them down and realize that I haven't seen Dave this morning.

"Is it nerve pain?" my mom interrupts my thoughts.

"Did Dave go home?" I blurt out. My mom studies me for a second and then replies with a simple, "Yes."

Good. I think to myself. *One less thing to deal with.*

Our conversation is interrupted when the pain in my stomach and the pressure on my tailbone are worsening.

My mom dials my in-home healthcare nurse's number and explains the situation to her. She recommends we hold tight and promises to get there right away to administer an enema. The pain in my stomach is excruciating. Out of desperation, my mom arranges two pillows beneath me in a makeshift donut shape to try to relieve some of the pressure. Beads of sweat form on my forehead from the exertion of pain management. I collapse into my bed as the nurse enters my room, carrying an enema kit. It's been well over a week since I've had a bowel movement.

"I'm sorry you're in pain," she says to me sympathetically. "Let's get you some relief. First, I'll turn you slightly onto your side to administer the enema, then we'll wheel you to the bathroom so you can relieve yourself." This is the one time I'm actually permitted to tilt onto my left side, propped up by a couple of pillows. At this point, any semblance of dignity has gone out the window. I've reached a stage where invasive treatments like enemas don't faze me anymore; I'm so desperate for relief, I don't care if the whole world is watching. As the nurse prepares the enema, I think back to my time in the hospital, where I went two weeks without one bowel movement. Nurses would delicately maneuver me onto my left side, perform the enema inducing movement, and then slip a small bedpan beneath me before returning me to my original position. Back then, I wasn't able to use a toilet chair yet, and the entire process was agonizing—I screamed through most of it.

As Shannon administers the saline solution into my body, I know relief is just around the corner. She then reclines me into an upright position and slowly inches me into my wheelchair.

Hurry up. I can't hold it much longer.

Finally, we reach the medical toilet bench. A wave of relief comes over me as I evacuate my bowels. Shannon is there, keeping watch, making sure I am okay, and then expertly guides me back to my hospital bed.

"I can't thank you enough for your help today," I express gratefully.

"It's my pleasure," Shannon replies warmly before heading out the door.

"I don't work on the weekends, so I'll see you on Monday," she adds.

Mom slips into my room quietly. "Feeling better, Cait?"

"Yeah . . . I am," I whisper, not feeling up for a conversation.

"You need anything?" she asks.

"Just a shower, Mom. That's all I want today." It has been days since my last shower, and I was starting to notice my own stench.

"You got it," my mom responds, promptly fetching my wheelchair.

Mom wheels me into the bathroom and assists me in undressing while I remain seated in my wheelchair. Carefully, she encases my pink leg cast in several layers of white garbage bags, securing them tightly with tape. With practiced hands, she guides me to the edge of the shower and helps me transfer to the shower bench. It's a complicated process, requiring both skill and effort, but thankfully, I still have the use of my arms to assist in stabilizing myself.

I tentatively reach for the hose, realizing it's the first time I've attempted to bathe myself since the accident. Previously, even the slightest movements would send waves of pain through my body, but now, with careful and deliberate motions, I feel confident that I can manage. The warm water soothes me so much that I find myself unconcerned about the fact that I can't even shave my hairy legs.

I ask my mom to leave me, and I linger for a while in the shower.

My last conversation with Dave enters my thoughts. *No, don't go there,* I think. *I'm not letting him ruin this moment of bliss.*

As the warm water continues to drip down my battered and broken body, I try to ignore all the thoughts swirling in my head for now and just savor the moment.

I hear a soft knock at the door.

"Cait, are you ready to get out?" my mom asks.

"Just a few more minutes," I respond.

"Dave's been trying to reach you. He's called three times."

My moment of uninterrupted bliss has been hijacked by him.

I brace myself for the inevitable conversation with Dave. I know how it will unfold— he'll apologize, express remorse, and try to tug at my heartstrings as he always does. *How long will I continue to play his game?*

I gaze down at the reddish-purple colored scar stretching a foot long over my abdomen, weaving its way across my back, and I am suddenly hit with a memory of visiting an art exhibit in college and learning about the famous Mexican painter Frida Kahlo. I was struck by her raw and graphic self-portrait paintings—I had never seen anything like them. I have a tendency to become fixated on certain individuals I find interesting, which left me spending hours reading about her remarkable, yet tragic life. The bus accident she endured left her physically shattered, but it was her marriage to Diego that truly left her broken and struggling to piece herself back together.

As I contemplate my future, it becomes increasingly clear that Dave doesn't have a place in it. His presence has become a source of nothing but negativity and pain, fueling my anxiety whenever he's nearby. The urge to protect myself intensifies as I realize the depth of trauma I've already endured, with the knowledge that more challenges await. I know I need to remove him from the equation entirely. Only then can I pave the way for healing to begin.

NINE

TONGUE DEPRESSORS
AND A HAPPY FACE

S pring has arrived. As I sit by the window, watching the world
bloom in all its fullness of color and life from the confines of
my wheelchair, I feel empty. The veil of denial that has been keeping
me alive has lifted, and I'm now forced to confront the stark reality
of my new normal. I should be gearing up for college graduation,
planning adventures with friends, yet here I am, grappling with
the weight of this truth—my new reality. A reality devoid of the
freedom I once took for granted. I'm a prisoner in my own body. It
hits me hard, the profound sense of loss, knocking me off balance
and leaving me disoriented and hollow.

Dave's persistent attempts to reach out go unanswered, each
call blocked without hesitation. However, his mother calls more

frequently than usual expressing genuine concern for my well-being. We talk about my recovery, the spring flowers, and what I'm watching on TV, every conversation avoiding the unspoken question hanging in the air—Dave. I am certain he has informed her of my decision to ignore his calls. The subtle probing about my emotional state confirms my suspicions. For now, I am grateful to avoid the elephant in the room.

A knock at the front door interrupts the quiet of my thoughts. Mom rushes to the door to greet our visitor.

I hear her welcome the knocker, and then her voice is directed at me. "Cait, your new therapist is here!" Her voice carries through the house, pulling me from my thoughts about Dave and his mom.

I groan as I shift uncomfortably in my wheelchair. I'm not up for therapy. My mood hovers low. For now, I am tethered to home-based sessions for the next couple of months before transitioning to site-based therapy. My surgeon explained to us that my body isn't ready for the back-and-forth journey to and from therapy multiple times a week.

I look up to see a woman about my mom's age walking toward me. She strikes an unassuming figure—of average height, slender, with tousled brown hair pulled back into a ponytail. Dressed in dark blue scrubs and tan Crocs, she exudes a sense of comfort and professionalism. "Hi, I'm Melissa," she says with a soft smile.

Mom spins my wheelchair around to face her, and as Melissa lays eyes on me for the first time, she lets out an involuntary gasp. Instantly, she tries to recover, realizing her misstep.

I quickly introduce myself as I try to brush off her reaction, having already grown accustomed to these kinds of responses from friends and family members.

It's not hard to guess why she reacted the way she did. These past few days have been a rough patch—filled with pain, sleepless nights, and a stubborn refusal to eat thanks to unbearable levels of nerve pain. I'm a shadow of my former self, my body is wasting away, deep bags have hollowed out the youthful light in my eyes, and my hair is layer upon layer of tangled and unkempt knots.

"Where would you like to set up for therapy?" she asks quickly, trying to regain her composure and resume the reason she is here in the first place. "I know you need to be lying down, and that you're in a hospital bed, but I think it would be easier if we tried our work in a regular bed," Melissa suggests.

"We have a guest room with a queen bed. We could try that," I suggest. I'm surprised at the relief I feel at the possibility of a change of scenery.

"I'll leave you two to tackle therapy. Let me know if there is anything you need." My mom excuses herself.

As Melissa wheels me into the guest bedroom, I feel a twinge of apprehension creeping in. I don't know anything about this therapist. And that means she knows nothing about me.

Surely, someone has briefed Melissa on my medical background by now?

We reach the edge of the bed, and as I take in the soft quilt draped over the queen-sized mattress, it dawns on me, I haven't lain in a regular bed in over two months. Every hospital bed I've encountered has been equipped with an incline feature, accommodating the strain on my pelvis area that prevents me from lying flat.

Melissa leans in to assist me out of my wheelchair, but I instinctively hold up a hand, halting her in her tracks. Her eyes widen momentarily, surprised by my abruptness.

"Is everything okay?" she asks quickly, straightening up.

"I'd just like to quickly go over my medical history first, if that's alright with you," I explain, attempting to smooth over the interruption with a half-hearted smile.

"Well, I've got it all here," Melissa responds, pulling a manilla file folder filled with my medical paperwork.

"Okay . . . well, I'd like to add a few things that might not be included there, if that's all right with you."

Melissa nods, acknowledging my request.

I delve into my medical history, starting with the frog-in-the-blender analogy that has become my go-to explanation. Melissa listens attentively, her eyebrows rising in surprise but otherwise unfazed by my candid remarks and vivid descriptions.

"I can't lay flat, so I'll need pillows to prop me up," I mention, hoping to preempt any discomfort.

Melissa springs into action, constructing a veritable fortress of pillows for me to lean against in the guest bed. With careful precision, she lifts me from the wheelchair and positions me on the bed. But as I sink into the mattress, the pressure bearing down on my tailbone starts to radiate pain.

"I don't know how long I can tolerate this for," the evident strain in my voice indicating my growing level of discomfort. "Did you take your pain medication today?" Melissa asks as she surveys my positioning, considering how to alleviate the added pressure. "Yes, I did," I choke out between breaths that are growing more and more shallow.

"Okay, we'll take it slow, and you let me know if you're uncomfortable at any time," she reassures me as she reaches for my paperwork.

I'm uncomfortable all the time, I want to scream.

"Let's start by gently bending your right knee into your chest," she suggests as she places my medical file on the chair next to the bed. My muscles clench instantly, memories of trauma flooding back as I recall movements that felt more like torture. Up until this point, my leg has only been slowly moved up a few inches and back down under the guidance of a physical therapist who knew my injuries inside and out. Initially, the pink-plaster cast extended from my midthigh to my foot, keeping my leg completely immobile. But after weeks of healing, it has been replaced with a partial cast, allowing for limited movement. Even so, it has been over two months since my right knee has seen anything close to a ninety-degree angle. Not to mention, my sciatic nerve was severed during one of my surgeries.

"Let's just take it very slowly," I respond slowly, trying to convey my fear.

"We'll take it easy, but we gotta get those joints moving," Melissa insists with the assurance of an expert who has been there, done that.

Melissa places one hand under my right leg, still encased in its bubble gum pink cast. Then, in one fluid motion, she forcefully pushes my knee toward my chest. I let out a scream as excruciating pain floods my body. It feels like my leg is being ripped right off my body and instinctively, I lash out, striking her in the chest with my fist, as I scream out again. The shock on her face mirrors my own, as my leg drops back onto the bed, only exacerbating the pain.

"What are you doing?!" I shout at her in frustration.

Taking a moment to catch my breath, I notice Melissa's gone silent, the weight of the situation sinking in as she tries to make sense of what just went down.

Wow. I actually hit her.

Simultaneously, apologies flow freely from both of us.

"We'll proceed much more gently from now on," she assures me, continuing to apologize throughout our session.

By the end of our time together, we're sharing laughter over the unexpected incident. "Next time, I'll come prepared with body armor," Melissa jokes on her way out.

* * *

This week, our home feels like a revolving door—with friends, family, and church members dropping in more than usual. While

I appreciate the company, socializing drains me in a way it never did before the accident. I've hit a point where I'm hesitant to say yes to any more invites, with the exception of close friends and family members. It's exhausting to plaster on a happy face every time someone knocks on the door. I've even started timing my pain meds to coincide with their visits, so I am able to continue masking the true extent of my suffering.

When I am asked the usual questions "How are you?" and "How are you feeling?" I find myself giving canned responses that couldn't be further from the truth. "I'm doing well," or "I'm tough, I'll pull through," are replied with practiced politeness. I understand their good intentions, but the repetition of clichés like "God won't give you more than you can handle" or "Just take it one day at a time" only compound my frustration.

Truth is, I'm really not okay. How could I be? My body feels like it has been through a meat grinder, and given the doctor's summaries, that is pretty accurate. There are moments when I just want to scream at everyone and their empty platitudes. I want to somehow convey the severity of my situation to them. Instead of forcing a smile and saying, "Everything happens for a reason!" through my wired teeth, I want to weep into my hands and tell the truth: Some days, it feels like I'm barely holding on. As I continue to lie for their benefit, I start to wonder how honesty came to feel so taboo, despite being a natural reaction to my circumstances. As I would half-listen to the updates in their lives, I wondered how they would react if, when it was my turn, I told them that, just a few days prior, I was literally tearing my hair out of my head from pain. Imagining their reaction, and the gossip that would ensue, I do my best to maintain a façade that everything is okay.

Why does it matter so much to me what others think? I consider as I float off into a medication-induced break from my pain.

My train of thought derails abruptly as the shrill ring of our house phone pierces the air, persistent and unrelenting; it doesn't stop.

Annoyed at the interruption to my self-loathing thoughts, I yell out, "Is anyone going to pick that up?"

Minutes stretch on, each ring a jarring interruption.

Finally, my mom enters my room, phone clutched in hand. Her weary face says it all.

"I know you said you're not up for any more visitors today, but Sue McCarthy won't stop calling. She and her daughter are eager to drop by," she explains, resigned.

I can feel an irritation bubbling up as I roll my eyes in response.

"Cait, I know you don't care for them. Frankly, neither do I, but they mean well, and they won't stop calling," she reassures me.

"I just can't handle loud voices, and I'd rather not be the subject of their town gossip. That's all they want—to get the latest scoop." I look at my mom, pleading for her to understand and communicate my message to them.

"I understand. I won't answer," she assures me.

I don't have the energy—or patience—to contend with the antics of the dynamic mother-daughter duo. Besides, I want to conserve my energy for tomorrow when two of my closest friends are coming to spend the day with me.

As the sun starts to go down, I sink back into the pillows of my hospital bed. Mom pops her head in once more, announcing her plans to prepare dinner before disappearing again. My pain levels begin to spike. With over an hour until my next dose of meds, I try to distract myself by filling the pages of the new journal I was gifted by a friend.

Just as I finish jotting down my thoughts, a knock at the front door shatters the quiet solitude I had cultivated with my writing. My heart sinks because it knows.

Oh no, not now.

Mom dutifully walks to the front door and answers it. My pain takes another stab at me as the boisterous voices of two distinctly Southern women echo through the house. I cover my face with my hands. Their footsteps draw closer, and I quickly pull the white sheet over myself, feeling exposed in my nightgown and my pain.

Without warning, two women barge into my room, the decibel of their voices overwhelming. Mom trails behind them, offering silent apologies with a helpless look in her eyes. Before I can even utter a greeting, the daughter scrutinizes me, her words a mix of surprise and awkward flattery.

"I thought your face was shattered. I guess I expected it to look worse, based on what I heard," she blurts out. Well, how's that for a hello.

My face was *shattered and reconstructed*, I defy her with my thoughts.

I awkwardly stare blankly at her, taken aback by her comment. I have nothing to say.

The interrogation begins without pause, and I realize quickly I am a wild animal trapped in a zoo, subject to their scrutiny, and whatever they want to carry back to town with them: "How are you?" "How long is your recovery?" "What caused the accident?" Their questions bombard me, one after the other, they don't come up for air, and certainly do not leave me with any room to respond. Mom and I exchange uncomfortable glances, silently willing them to wrap it up.

As the conversation shifts to their own lives, I find a moment of relief from the spotlight. Yet, the chatter continues unabated, stretching on for what feels like an eternity. My pain intensifies, and mom steps in, gracefully ending the visit.

"I think Cait has reached her limit, and we need to let her rest."

Awkward glances pass between Sue and her daughter as they say their goodbyes, leaving me drained and fighting pain. Mom returns to find me in tears, my sheets soaked with sweat and my body trembling from the pain their intensity has caused. She hands me a bottle of oxycodone. I gratefully pop the pills in my mouth as I tightly clutch my pillow.

It's only after the medication kicks in that I can speak again. "We need to be more careful about visitors, Mom," I manage to say.

"I had no idea they would show up like that, let alone behave so . . . inappropriately," she admits, apologetically.

"That's just how they are. Unfortunately, everyone in town knows it," I reply.

I skip dinner. All I can think about now is closing my eyes. Tonight is the first night since returning home that I effortlessly drift off to sleep and manage to stay that way through the night without any interruptions.

Morning quickly approaches and with it something I've been looking forward to—a visit from my childhood best friends. As we reminisce and catch up, I recount the unexpected visit from the previous night.

"The audacity of her to broadcast her time with you on social media," Kim vents, rolling her eyes.

"And what she said about your face . . ." Leah went on, still stunned by the inappropriate remark.

True to their nature, my friends are fiercely loyal and protective. Without hesitation, Kim whips out her cell phone and dials Sue's daughter who had intruded on us. She delivers a stern message, asserting that any future visits must be pre-approved by her. I can't help but laugh and shake my head in amusement. Kim and I share a deep history, and she is notorious for having my back. I'm so grateful to see that while my life has been upended, at least this one thing hasn't changed.

*   *   *

The weeks crawl by, each day feeling longer than the last. It's like living in my own version of *Groundhog Day*, where I am stuck in this endless loop of routine: wake up, mom helps me dress, I pop pain pills, shift from bed to wheelchair throughout the day, go to restless sleep at night, repeat. While I've managed to venture out in my wheelchair on occasion to soak up the warmth of the sun, the joy is always short-lived as pain forces me back indoors and back into my hospital bed.

Today, I'm scheduled for surgery to remove the wires clamping my jaw shut. The prospect of facing yet another surgery makes me want to vomit, yet I know it's necessary for me to regain normal eating habits. And with my mouth wired shut, I couldn't vomit easily anyway! Mom enters my room. We're in a rush to make it to my pre-op appointment, but everything moves slowly these days. A profound exhaustion has taken root and seems here to stay accompanied by unyielding pain. I feel so weak and frail.

"Where are your pants?" Mom's question snaps me back to reality, realizing both pairs of oversized black pants that I alternate into are in the dirty laundry. Panic sets in as I realize I'm left with no other options. My clothing choices are limited because of the swelling and pain, especially in the lower half of my body.

"Dirty pants it is," I say with a sigh, resigned to making do with what's available.

Mom helps me into my clothes, and Dad has the car ready to go. It's my first time in a vehicle, other than the ambulance ride home, since before the accident. Once I am fully dressed—dirty black pants and all—mom wheels me to the passenger side. As Dad assists me into the car, I feel strange sitting upright instead of reclined in my wheelchair. With a deep breath, I brace myself for the discomfort ahead.

I swallow down another dose of painkillers to stay ahead of the pain while Dad tries to lighten the mood with his jokes during our journey to the hospital. Around twenty minutes into the drive, a wave of intense fire-like pain radiates from my tailbone down to my feet. Desperately, I try to alleviate the pressure, gripping onto the door and the center console for support. With just ten minutes to go, I shift my focus to the outside world passing by. I'm suddenly hit with an overwhelming grief and clarity that I can never unsee; my old life—goals and dreams, superficial relationships that didn't really matter, material possessions that were not important—it all suddenly becomes meaningless when your quality of life is compromised. My health now matters to me more than ever before because I see how fleeting it can be.

I think about the way I have been met with so much love and grace from my family, close friends, and the medical community, which has made my situation bearable. It's enough to bring me to tears right there in the front seat of my parents' car because here's the thing about recovering from serious injuries—it's not just the pain in your body that you experience, it's painfully isolating for your heart. Your body, mind, heart, and soul desperately want to move backward in time—to recoup what has been lost. The problem is, everything and everyone else continues to move forward—with or without you—like being a passenger on a bus, watching the world go by, you are headed in a direction you can't control and know nothing about, and everyone else out there continues to carry on. I feel this overwhelming urge to break through the window and scream at the entire world to stop—to beg them to look at me, to hold me, to *just stop!*

"We're here," Dad announces our arrival to the surgical facility, interrupting my thoughts.

I swallow back the lump in my throat. "Yep, let's get this show on the road," I respond, as I wipe tears from my eyes.

"You'll do great," he reassures, helping me into my wheelchair.

Having already endured a marathon sixteen-hour surgery and subsequent procedures, I try to convince myself that this one will be a breeze.

My parents wheel me into the hospital and I'm met with warmth and kindness from the nurses and staff. They waste no time preparing me for the procedure, which I appreciate amidst my rising anxiety.

"Everything's going to be fine, Cait. We'll be waiting right here for you," Mom and Dad reassure me as I am wheeled through heavy doors.

The thought of uncovering my teeth, which have been hidden under wires for months, hasn't crossed my mind until now. Before I can dwell on it, the anesthesiologist comes in. "Okay, you're about to take a little nap. We'll take good care of you," he says, and with that, everything fades to black.

*   *   *

I slowly regain consciousness nearly four hours later, greeted by a metallic taste of blood in my mouth. The surgery is over. All the wires have been successfully removed.

A nurse swiftly places a large piece of white gauze in my mouth to stem the bleeding. I feel groggy, and struggle to form coherent sentences. Mom and Dad enter my room. Dad reaches for my hand, squeezing it tightly, Mom tenderly strokes my head.

My oral surgeon Dr. Dean strides into the room to check on me. "You did great! Your teeth look fantastic, no signs of decay. We managed to clean them up for you while you were asleep. It seems like you took good care of them while the wires were in," he praises. I attempt to respond, but my words come out slurred as I drift in and out of consciousness.

"Don't worry about talking right now; there will be plenty of time for that soon," Dr. Dean assures me before turning to my parents. "It'll still be a couple of weeks before Caitlin can handle solid foods," he informs them.

Mom nods, processing the information, as Dr. Dean places a large bag of tongue depressors on the table next to my bed. "These will be used to open Caitlin's jaws slowly over time. Here are detailed instructions on how to proceed," he explains, handing the paperwork to my mom.

"Pry her mouth open?" my mom asks skeptically.

"Yes, essentially. She'll stack the tongue depressors on top of each other, adding a new one every two days. She'll need to keep them stacked in her mouth for several minutes multiple times a day. After about two weeks, she can start with soft, solid foods," Dr. Dean clarifies.

"Okay, we'll go over the directions with Caitlin once she's fully conscious," Mom agrees.

After another hour in post-op, I finally awaken fully. My mouth is swollen and my gums are throbbing from where the wires were removed, but despite the pain, all I can think about is food.

"When can I eat again?" I blurt out.

"Your surgeon said it'll be another two weeks," my dad says.

The disappointment weighs heavy. The desire to eat real food is more intense than ever. I'm in pain, but I'm hungry too.

My parents assist me into my wheelchair, my mouth packed with white gauze. During the car ride, my dad glances over to see blood and drool trickling down the side of my mouth. Oblivious to it all, I have lost all sensation on the right side of my jaw and part of my face due to nerve damage. Numb from the extra painkillers, I am asleep for most of the ride.

I drift in and out of sleep throughout the day and well into the night, only to be jolted awake by waves of agonizing pain coursing through my jaw and every inch of my body.

"There's not a single spot that doesn't hurt like hell right now, Mom," I groan.

In response, my mom retrieves several bags of frozen peas, strategically placing them on different areas of my body. Little do I realize; this ritual marks just the beginning of many nights where frozen peas become my unlikely allies in battling sleeplessness and relentless pain. Wide eyed and restless, I find myself unable to go back to sleep.

*　　*　　*

It's morning time. *Finally.* The light filtering through my bedroom window gives me a sense of relief, somehow knowing that the long night has finally come to an end brings me peace. Nights have become something I dread, in the dark and quiet I'm alone in my hospital bed left to grapple with feelings of fear and loneliness while the ever-present excruciating pain radiates through my body. Morning never comes quickly enough.

Mom knocks on my door and enters with a couple of Ensure drinks, placing them on my nightstand. Though the wires that once held my mouth shut are removed, I still can't open my mouth fully.

My jaw feels trapped, as if it's resisting any attempt to move. It's a strange sensation that I struggle to adapt to. Not to mention my red and inflamed gums that once hosted the wires now burn and throb. I reach for the chocolate nutrition drink and take a small sip. I want to gag. I'm done with this liquid diet!

"Can you pass me the bag of tongue depressors, please?" I ask, ready to take on the challenge despite the early hour and the heaviness of fatigue lingering from a sleepless night.

My mom, ever the voice of reason, hesitates, "Do you really want to start now? You've barely had a moment to wake up, let alone prepare for the day."

"I've spent most of the night staring at the ceiling. I need to feel like I'm doing something productive," I insist.

Handing me the bag of jumbo-sized tongue depressors, my mom reads aloud the instructions for our unconventional morning routine. "Day one: Insert one tongue depressor into the mouth and hold for five minutes. Repeat every thirty minutes or as tolerated."

"This is crazy," I mutter under my breath, overwhelmed by the prospect.

I carefully attempt to insert the wooden stick into my mouth, but a jolt of pain shoots from the sides of my jaw to my ears. I push through until I manage to wedge the tongue depressor between my teeth, barely prying my mouth open. I motion for my mom to start the timer. As the minutes drag on, I'm reminded not only of the pain in my jaw but of the relentless ache that permeates a large portion of my body. I feel a blend of anger and frustration course through me. I don't want anything to do with these damn wooden sticks. It's relentless, layer upon layer of pain pressing down, suffocating me. All I want is to escape back to the life I once knew, to find some sense of normalcy. But deep down, reality sinks its teeth into me like I long to do with my own teeth on the tongue depressors—there's no way back to that girl. She was gone the moment she was projected through the windshield of that car at 90 miles per hour. My temples throb with tension as my hands instinctively find their way there, a telltale sign of my mounting frustration. I feel tears pricking at the corners of my eyes just as the familiar roar of a car engine outside my window shatters the fragile peace.

Dave.

TEN

"STOP FEELING SORRY FOR YOURSELF"

The roar of his black Audi's engine startles me. My muscles contract and I ease the tongue depressor out, fumbling to place it on my nightstand beside my stack of painkillers. I carefully touch my jaw, still feeling the discomfort caused by my recent surgery. I had this feeling that Dave would show up unannounced, as usual. But then, I had made sure his mom knew the date, knowing she'd tell him. Part of me wanted him to know. *Here I am, enduring another surgery because of his reckless actions. Here I am, battling more pain and now forced to pry my mouth open with these stupid tongue depressors.*

It's been weeks since we last spoke, yet I still find myself trapped in a torturous cycle of wanting him by my side while knowing he's incapable of being the partner I deserve. The trauma of the accident binds us in a way I can't fully comprehend, complicating my already tangled emotions. A part of me wants to scream at him and tell him to get off my property. At the same time, the vulnerable side of me yearns for him to step up, own his faults, and help me navigate this recovery. But I know that will never happen. That's just not Dave.

I hear another vehicle pull up in the driveway and recognize the voices of my uncle and cousins. They're probably here to talk to my dad about sports or fishing, as they often do. Moments later, my sister bursts through my bedroom door, red-faced and looking disheveled.

"Dave is . . ." She tries to get the words out, but I cut her off.

"Yeah . . . I know."

"Did you know he was coming?" she asks, accusation in her eyes.

"I had a feeling he would show up. Plus, I can recognize the sound of his engine anywhere."

"Uncle Tom just arrived with the kids, and they're chatting with Dave. You won't believe what he said—Dave scolded Austin for leaning against his car, asking if he would wash his fingerprints off! You could tell it bothered Uncle Tom," my sister exclaimed.

I roll my eyes. "Seriously? Austin is only six."

We hear the front door open, and my mom greets Dave as she lets him in. True to form, my sister bolts out of my bedroom. "I'm out of here. I have nothing to say to that asshole."

She is never one to stick around for drama.

I quickly grab the remote attached to my hospital bed to elevate it to an upright position. Anxiously, I run my fingers through my tangled hair, trying to look somewhat presentable.

Oh, who cares? I'm done trying to impress him.

Dave steps into my room, eyebrows raised beneath a red, flat-billed hat. The strong scent of high-end men's cologne fills the air, a signature of his taste for the best. Without a word, he closes the door behind him. His gaze feels heavy on me, silently judging. I know he's itching to comment on how bad I look or to tell me I need to push harder in my recovery. Folding my arms across my chest, in silent self-defense, I shift to find a comfortable position in the hospital bed.

"Hi," I manage, glancing in his direction.

"Hi," he replies, approaching my bed. "Well, old metal mouth is no more," he jokes, noticing the wires are gone from my mouth.

"Why are you here? Just to insult me again?" I snap.

"I'm here to be with you. My mom said you just had surgery, and I wanted to check on you."

"Well, I'm home and I'm fine," I respond sharply looking toward the door.

"You don't look fine. And . . . I just want you to get back to your old self again," he hazards.

"And you think I don't want that? That I don't pray for that every single day?" I feel my body starting to tremble with the injustice of it all.

"Praying is not going to get you out of this situation," he spats back.

"How would you know? You've never prayed a day in your life."

Dave glances at his phone, his attention divided between our conversation and his device. "If I was in your situation, I think I'd just off myself."

Did he really just say that? I roll my eyes and let out a seething breath between my unwired teeth.

"You know—you've never truly faced anything hard in your life. Everything has come easy, handed to you on a silver platter! You've never endured a life-altering ordeal that strips away your health and sense of self! You've never felt the agony of drifting off to sleep with your bones feeling as if they're being crushed repeatedly. I can't dress myself, shower, or even use the bathroom without assistance. Every shred of my dignity has been taken from me!"

Dave tilts his head down. I sense the storm brewing within him. By now, I am well acquainted with the triggers that set him off, and I refuse to hold back any longer. Without a single word, he turns and leaves the room, his footsteps echoing through the house until the finality of the front door's slam.

Maybe he's just stepping outside for a bit.

Moments later, my sister and mom burst into my room. "What happened? He was here for five minutes and is now strolling down the street?" my mom asks.

"Yep, he's taking a breather, I suppose," I reply much more nonchalantly than I feel.

"What did you say?" my mom inquires.

"All the right things," I reply, shifting to find another more comfortable position. All this drama is making my head hurt.

"Cait, maybe it's time to let go and move forward. You two can't even be in the same room for five minutes without clashing," Mom suggests gently.

"There's a part of me that hates him. But I don't know how to break free from him," I answer, my voice cracking as I stare out the window.

My mom and sister sit quietly. No one knows what to say.

Awkwardly, I change the subject. "I guess I'll freshen up while he's away. I feel so filthy."

Mom helps me into my wheelchair and wheels me to the bathroom. No shower today, just a quick wipe-down with wet wipes. I tie my hair back, dab on some cherry ChapStick, apply deodorant, and then Mom helps me back into my hospital bed.

Dave returns half an hour later, and neither of us discusses the argument that took place earlier. "Where did you disappear to?" I ask.

"Just needed some air," he replies.

"So what are the wooden sticks for anyway?" he asks casually, pointing to the stack of tongue depressors on the nightstand.

"To pry open my mouth. My doctor said it could take a couple of weeks."

"What the hell?" he exclaims.

"Yeah, it's fun," I quip sarcastically. "But it's the only way I'll be able to eat solid foods again, so I don't have a choice."

"Want to get out of this room? I could take you outside for a bit," he offers, his gaze softening as he takes in the whole picture of what I have become.

I agree as Dave awkwardly helps me into my wheelchair, clearly inexperienced with the task. I immediately tense up, bracing for the pain that movement inevitably brings. There's no way around it.

He navigates me through the house and out the garage door onto the wheelchair ramp. I feel my mom and sister's eyes on us. I give them an awkward thumbs-up to signal that everything is okay. Dave rolls me up and down the driveway a few times. At one point, he stops and stares in the direction of my parents' home, lost in thought for what feels like several minutes.

"What's wrong?" I ask.

"Oh, nothing," he responds.

"Obviously, it's something. You're just awkwardly staring."

Dave clears his throat. "We just come from two different worlds," he replies, shaking his head.

"What is that supposed to mean?"

"Don't worry about it," he cuts me off and starts to push me again.

No. You're not getting off that easy.

"You just think you're so much better than me and my family," I respond sharply—it's more of an accusation than anything.

Dave hesitates, as if about to reply, then swiftly wheels me back into the house, seemingly trying to avoid another argument.

My voice rises, fueled by the rage that has been boiling up inside me. "Look, if you're too good to stay here, then just leave. If you want to offer your 'support,' I would prefer you do it from afar! There's a hotel down the road—though it probably won't meet your standards."

We enter my bedroom and Dave pushes my wheelchair up to the edge of my hospital bed, and helps me into bed. He is, once again, head down, absorbed in his phone, uninterested in anything I have to say. Obviously, he couldn't care less and doesn't even want to be here.

Why does he keep coming back? Why won't he just break it off with me?

Silently, he turns toward the door, leaving without so much as a goodbye. My sister rushes in, eyes wide with questions. "Is he leaving? Did you break up with him?"

"I told him to go stay at a hotel," I reply.

"What? Why?" she asks, clearly puzzled.

"It doesn't matter, Ash. I just don't want him staying in our home."

"When will he be back?"

"Who knows!"

"He's such a jerk. You deserve so much better, Cait."

"Thanks," I mutter as she closes the door behind her.

Seething with anger, I feel that familiar trapped sensation come over me. It hits me like a direct punch in the gut. I grab my pillow and scream into it, sobbing.

"How did I get here?!" I cry out, expecting some divine answer from above. Instead, I am met with silence.

After what felt like an ample amount of time to commit to my pity party, I grab the large bag of tongue depressors off my bedside table, reluctantly reach inside and pull out two sticks. I insert the first one, barely prying my mouth open. The pain is tolerable this time. Progress.

I attempt to place another stick on top of the one snugly fitted inside my mouth. No chance. Frustration wells up inside me and I have the urge to manually pry my mouth open with my hands, just to get it over with. I try once more, but it's no use. I need more time. And time is one thing I have in abundance these days.

The next day feels like any other, monotonous and predictable. Then the phone rings. . . . It's a nurse from Summit Hospital in Texas, calling to inform my parents that it's time for me to wean off the fentanyl pain patch. The instructions are sparse.

"The withdrawal process will not be easy, but it's time for Caitlin to get off of it and just continue with other painkillers," the nurse explains.

"How do I 'wean' off a pain patch?" I ask my parents.

"I don't know," Mom replies. "They didn't really give us clear instructions. They just said to stop using it. Should we try cutting the patches in half?"

Dad rubs his head, clearly deep in thought. "Let me give Dave a call at the pharmacy, just to be safe."

Dad phones and the conversation is brief. I notice a concerned look on his face.

"He said do *not* cut the patches," Dad reports. "Because it's time-released, cutting it would cause all the medication to enter your system at once, possibly killing you."

Mom's eyes widen. "Thank God you called," she says.

Before my accident, I had never taken painkillers, aside from the occasional ibuprofen for a hormone-induced headache. I certainly had no idea about medication withdrawal and neither did my parents.

"Well, should we go ahead and remove the patch now?" Mom asks.

"Yeah, why not," I respond, completely oblivious to the horror that awaits me.

Mom makes her way over and helps me shift to the edge of the hospital bed, my legs dangling off. She assists as I remove my nightgown and then gently peels the sticky, white patch off me. It's odd to have it gone—the patch has been on my body for months now; it's almost as if it has become a part of me.

"It's off. I guess now all we can do is wait and see what happens," mom says quietly.

I don't think much of it as she helps me back into bed. But as evening approaches, I notice myself becoming increasingly restless and agitated. Mom comes into my room with a dinner tray of mashed-up chicken and dumplings. I'm getting better at opening my mouth, but I still can't chew. The tongue depressors are helping some, but it's an annoyingly slow process when trying to pry open a jaw that has been stuck in one position for months.

Mom sets the tray down on my nightstand. The clang of the tray hitting the table feels like a jolt of lightning hits my brain. I immediately put my hands to my ears and close my eyes to block everything out.

"Your face looks pale," she observes, placing her hand on my forehead. "Are you feeling okay?"

"Just really agitated and restless," I snap.

"I wonder if this is a side effect of not having the medication."

"I'm really not hungry and I just don't want to hear anyone talk right now," I respond, putting a pillow over my face.

"I'm worried about you. Just call me on the house phone if you need anything."

I nod in response, still under the pillow. Mom steps out of the room and I pull the pillow down over my chest and hug it tightly. Taking a deep breath, I drift off to sleep.

It's 7:00 p.m. and I awake abruptly, sheets soaked in sweat. I'm still clutching my pillow, my breathing heavy, my eyes painfully sensitive to the light. I shut them tightly, trying to find some relief.

Mom pokes her head into my room. "You look like you've seen a ghost," she remarks.

"I don't know what's wrong with me. Get Dad," I manage to say, my voice shaky.

My body starts shaking uncontrollably. "I need a blanket," I say, my teeth chattering. "It hurts to move, but the shaking won't stop!"

Tears well up in my eyes, and before I know it, I'm crying. Big, hot tears stream down my face, as loud, heart-wrenching sobs escape from deep inside me.

"What's happening? I feel like I'm going crazy!" I cry out.

Dad looks at me with deep sympathy, as if he understands. "It's the fentanyl," he says softly.

"What can we do?" Mom asks, panic overtaking her concern.

"It's just getting worse!" I scream.

"What's worse?" they ask in unison.

"I don't know! My body! Everything hurts," I sob.

I want so desperately to throw myself onto the floor, to toss and turn, curl up in a ball—anything to escape this agony. But I can't even rotate onto my side. I clutch the sweat-soaked sheets, my entire body cramping painfully, including my stomach. The cramps are relentless.

"I think I'm going to be sick," I gasp, as I press the incline button on my hospital bed.

Mom rushes out of the room and quickly returns with a large stainless steel mixing bowl. "This will have to do," she says, attempting to catch her breath. Dad grabs the bowl and shoves it into my lap just as vomit erupts from my mouth, splashing into the bowl, onto the sheets, and splattering onto his collared shirt. He doesn't move, just holds the bowl steady, his face tense with concern. In the background, I hear the sobs of my mom and sister who had slipped into the room unnoticed. The horror continues as more vomit pours out of me, and my body flushes with heat.

"Get this blanket off of me!" I plead, trying my best not to knock the bowl of vomit onto the floor. I feel like I am on fire and I'm terrified about what I'm going to feel next.

Dad yanks the soiled blanket and sheets away as Mom carefully removes the vomit-filled mixing bowl.

"Ash, go get towels and trash bags," Mom instructs.

I'm burning up, my body consumed by what feels like a raging fever and the worst flu of my life. I continue to shake uncontrollably as I thrash my head from side to side, desperate for relief.

"Call someone, Mike," my mom urges, "Is this even normal?"

Dad doesn't answer. But reaches for his phone and dials his local doctor friend. I can hear him talking on the phone explaining the situation, but his voice sounds like a distant echo. It no longer feels like I'm in my bedroom. *Am I back in the hospital?* I wonder as I shake and shutter with fever.

"The doctor said you may go through the blues," he says, as he looks in my direction.

"The blues!" my mom blurts out. "This is far from the blues, Mike."

"I'm freezing! I need a blanket," I blurt out. More shaking. Mom grabs a thick blanket and gently places it over me.

As the symptoms dial-up in intensity, my internal thermostat seems to go haywire. I am sweating profusely but when I glance down, I notice I am covered in goosebumps. Basic primal urges kick in, like the desperate need for food or water. I'll do anything to relieve this torment. There's a part of me that just wants to put the pain patch back on and make this nightmare go away. But I know I'll have to go through this hell all over again. Even within the haze of withdrawal, I know I have no choice but to ride it out.

At some point in the night, the truth hits me: my body is addicted to fentanyl.

This wasn't by choice. I had no other options—my survival depended on those patches. But why wasn't I informed about the dangers of these drugs or the horrific withdrawal symptoms that would follow when I tried to get off?

"I can't do this anymore!" I cry out, my sobs echoing in the room. Mom hugs me. Even her gentle touch makes me tense up. Dad and Ash bring dining room chairs into the room so they will have a place to sit and rest, signaling what we all know but don't want to say out loud: This is going to be a long night.

"I just want to die!" I scream. "How do we make it stop?" My parents, completely helpless, have shock written all over their faces. No one was prepared for this.

"Why didn't they tell me this would happen?" I sob.

"I don't know, Cait," Mom whispers, her voice trembling. "I really just don't know."

Ash takes a turn rubbing my head as it dangles off the side of the hospital bed. My body goes completely limp, only to start violently shaking minutes later.

Dave is nowhere to be found. *He's probably in his hotel room, indulging in the finest cuisine and playing Xbox,* I think to myself. Or maybe he left without telling anyone and traveled back home.

Mom and Dad are exhausted, so they rotate shifts to get some sleep. I desperately want to sleep. Sleep means escape from this withdrawal nightmare. Seconds feel like minutes, and minutes feel like hours. There's no reprieve. I try clenching my fists and tightening my entire body to relieve the restlessness, but I'm hit with a crushing pain throughout my pelvis.

"Mom," I whisper quietly, "I need oxycodone. Now."

Mom wakes up, startled. She staggers to her feet, still half-asleep, and reaches for the orange bottle of painkillers on the dresser, handing me one. I am hopeful the oxycodone will take the edge off the withdrawal symptoms, and it does. Not much, but I'll take even the slightest reprieve from the torment. It's at least enough for Mom to get a full hour of uninterrupted sleep.

Watching the clock and waiting for the morning is agonizingly slow. In my experience, pain and sickness always feel worse once the sun goes down.

Morning finally comes, and I pass out from sheer exhaustion. Mom quietly slips out of my room. I'm not sure how long I am asleep, but the reprieve from my suffering feels short-lived. I open my eyes and see a figure sitting next to me.

"Dave? I thought you went back to Texas," I say groggily.

"Nope, just thought it was best if I stayed away a little while and let things cool off. . . . Looks like not much has changed since I left," he remarks.

I look away toward the wall and don't respond immediately as my mind recalls the horrific events of the night before. I start breaking out in sweat again, clenching my fists to keep from yelling out in frustration. It occurs to me just how much the body and brain get used to having opioids around. It's as if my body snarls for medication, like a trapped tiger who has been starved for weeks.

Dave finally takes notice of my weary disposition.

"Everything okay?"

"*No*, everything is not *okay*. We removed the fentanyl patch yesterday, and now I am in full-blown withdrawal."

"Woah!" he says, leaning in closer to examine me as if I were a zoo animal on display. "What are your symptoms?" he asks, for once taking a slight interest in my case.

"Everything from sweating to vomiting and shaking. I feel like I am going crazy. Last night was hell."

"I know a guy who got addicted to fentanyl after just five days of use. You were on it for months. Are the docs not giving you anything to ease the symptoms?" he asks.

At this point, I can't tell if he is being sympathetic or just finds this sort of thing amusing.

"No. *No one* prepared me for this," I say as I begin to violently shake. "I didn't even receive basic care to manage the symptoms. Nothing."

"Wow," he responds.

Mom interrupts our conversation as she enters my room; she's completely exhausted. Dad follows close behind, both of them ignore Dave.

Dave manages a simple "Hi," but nothing else is said. Eventually, he excuses himself. "I'm headed out to grab lunch. I'll be back this evening."

"See you later," Mom replies, as I catch Dad rolling his eyes in annoyance.

For hours, I toss and turn, alternating between hot and cold. Mom washes my sweat-soaked sheets on and off throughout the day. Dad, Mom, and Ash take turns sitting with me.

"Take me to the ER or just give me a sedative and put me out of my misery. I can't do this anymore!" I plead.

No one says anything. Everyone is paralyzed by helplessness.

Dad has been researching like a madman online, looking up withdrawal symptoms and what to expect. "We just have to give it a few days," he responds, lightly touching the top of my leg.

"Days? No! I can't do days," I put my hands over my face, whimpering, pleading to them for relief.

"We will help you through this. You're not alone." It is meant as an assurance, but the fear is obvious as my mom moves from my bed to the dining room chair.

Sure enough, Dave arrives just as the sun goes down and sits next to my hospital bed. My parents exchange awkward glances and then leave the room to give us privacy.

We chat for a bit and then to my surprise, I burst into tears. "I was never told I could become dependent on these drugs! Never counseled. Nothing! It's not enough that I had to endure this accident, multiple surgeries, pain, isolation, my mouth wired shut, and now—THIS nightmare!" I continue to sob as I look to Dave for encouragement, sympathy . . . anything.

He just stares at me, quietly observing me like I am a science experiment.

"Aren't you going to say anything?" I groan.

He looks on for a few seconds longer, then reaches out and pats my head. "Just . . . I don't know . . . go to sleep and stop feeling sorry for yourself. You'll feel better in the morning."

Then, in one fluid motion, he rises from the chair, grabs his key fob out of his pocket, clicks the unlock button, and reaches for the doorknob. I hear the beep of his car unlocking. He's gone without another word or even so much as a glance back in my direction.

I lie there, staring at the ceiling that seems to stretch on forever, stunned by his response and lack of empathy. I can't even bring myself to lash out at him. He has already broken me, beaten me down until there is nothing left.

*　　*　　*

The withdrawals drag on for nearly two weeks, not just a few days like Google had promised my dad. I'm constantly drenched in sweat, gripped by a deep, unsettling jitteriness that keeps me twitching and writhing all night. The most disturbing part is the crying—sudden, uncontrollable sobbing overtakes me for no apparent reason. I'm stuck in a nightmare, and each day, the darkness closes in a little more. I barely eat or sleep, and daily habits like showering and brushing my teeth fall by the wayside. But the worst part is the depression; I am overwhelmed every minute of every day by this crushing sense of hopelessness. It's in those dark hours, in the middle of the night, when I am most alone, that I start to believe I will never recover.

Journal entry. Worse than pain is the loss of hope for health to return. Job 7:7

My brain struggles to adjust to life without fentanyl, and thoughts of dying frequently invade my mind. It's like an out-of-body experience that never ends. One minute I am having intrusive fantasies of a strange man dressed in a black trench coat breaking into my room and ending it all for me, and the next, I am hit with flashbacks to happy times from my childhood. I quietly cry out to God, begging for relief, for an end to this relentless torment.

I toss and turn in the night as more memories from my past surface. Pictures of my childhood, running barefoot through the woods, or lemonade stands at my grandparents' house visit me. I dream about the first moment my dad gifted me with my beloved hound dog Copper. One by one the most beautiful memories of my life play out before me like the scenes of a movie and the soundtrack is a familiar hymn I have grown up with, "It Is Well with My Soul." I start to whisper the lyrics quietly as I lay in bed. Enveloped in complete darkness, I whisper words penned a hundred years ago, and remember the heart-wrenching story behind its composure. The immense grief the composer must have felt after losing everything and then writing those words; I feel a strange connection to him as if I can somehow sense his pain. Then something miraculous happens—I drift off into a peaceful sleep.

Hours later, my eyes flicker open to the sun beaming in through my blinds. I brace myself for that dreaded feeling, the restlessness, the agitation, but surprisingly, there's nothing waiting for me this morning. Instead, I am met by the morning sun and a rare stillness. The monstrous grip of fentanyl is finally released. My symptoms are gone. Vanished. As if they were never there.

I continue to lay very still in bed for several minutes, waiting to be hit with another wave of more agonizing withdrawal symptoms as I try to process the roller coaster ride of the past two weeks. Still, nothing happens. However, a new pain unveils itself. While the withdrawal effects of the fentanyl have subsided, I am still living in a broken body. The holes in my jaw and mouth where the wires once were, throb. The herniated discs all throughout my back and neck and the newly formed scar tissue around my torn muscles pulse relentlessly. Sometimes, I picture my pain like the ocean I grew up next to, its waves crashing in unpredictable rhythms. One moment, it's the searing burn of nerve damage, lightning bolts coursing through severed pathways, looking for a part of my body to tether to. The next—it's a deep, bone-weary ache, as if my skeleton protests its own existence. There is no relief—only a shifting of the burden from one pain to the next.

Groggily, I reach for my orange pill bottle and pop an oxycodone into my mouth. I sleep on and off for most of the day, only waking to eat and drink. At some point, I ask my mom for a pen and sticky notes. With a tray on my lap, I start writing out the lyrics with a Sharpie marker to the song I had quietly sung to myself the night before. I then position them in a row on the wall beside my hospital bed. The words bring me comfort—knowing they were written by someone who had everything dear ripped from him, yet whose faith remained unshaken—he was proof that I could survive.

The withdrawal nightmare finally ends for me. Though I am weak, frail, and still very much in recovery, coming out of that ordeal gives me newfound strength and the faith to keep pressing forward.

If I can survive being thrown out of a car at 90 miles per hour and a fentanyl addiction—how much more could I overcome?

ELEVEN

STYROFOAM CUP

How did I get here?

I gaze down at my legs, my right ankle is throbbing beneath the pink cast, its shattered pieces determinedly healing back together inside. The pain and swelling are worse than usual; so intense that I want to rip the cast off my leg. Before the accident, my only experience with an injury was when I tore all the ligaments in my right ankle during a flag football game. I remember colliding with an opponent and feeling my ankle twist unnaturally. As I fell to the ground, pain seared through me, and I began tearing at the well-manicured grass in distress. A knock at my bedroom door breaks into my thoughts.

My dad waits for me to say "Come in!" before he slides the door open wide enough to stick his head into the room. "Do you want me to push you outside in your wheelchair for a bit?" Dad asks.

Wincing as my ankle pulses with pain, I answer. "I don't really feel up to it right now."

He studies me for a moment and then asks tentatively, "Everything okay?"

"Something is wrong with my ankle. There's so much pain and pressure!" I say through gritted teeth. "But I don't want to go to the ER and wait for hours. This feels too urgent."

Dad picks up on my anxiety immediately—we've been here before. "I'll phone Dr. Aston and ask if he can see you after hours. Hang tight, I'll be right back." Dr. Aston has been a family friend for as far back as I could remember, treating my dad and uncles for various athletic injuries over the years.

"We are good to go! Dr. Aston is going to meet us at his office in twenty minutes!" Dad announces, grabbing my wheelchair and pushing it toward my bed.

"What's going on?" My mom has now joined us, a dish towel in one hand, a plate in the other she must have been in the middle of drying. I can tell she is sensing that something is off.

"Everything is okay. Don't panic. We are just going to have Dr. Aston look at Cait's ankle. She says it's hurting worse than usual."

Mom rushes to the kitchen, grabs her purse from the countertop, and in less than two minutes, we are out the door. Dad carefully helps me into the car. The stabbing pain in my ankle is unbearable as I grip the sides of my seat to get through the nausea it brings.

It's a short five-minute drive to Dr. Aston's office, located in a solid red brick building I've passed countless times since childhood. Dad parks the car and wheels me to the door where Dr. Aston greets us warmly. Efficient in my distress, he leads us to the back of the clinic.

Dad and mom adeptly assist me up onto the exam table, but I'm too tormented to notice their skilled help with my damaged body, busy groaning to find some kind of release from this hell.

"Something is really wrong," I sob. "Please, take it off!" I'm begging now, desperation tinging my voice. Dr. Aston nods his head in agreement and tries his best to calm me down. He takes the cast saw and gently works the small-toothed blade through the plaster to liberate my leg. As he peels it off, his eyes widen when he examines my ankle.

As soon as the last piece of cast is peeled away from my leg, I feel relief. It's so visceral, like the relief that comes with a sudden release of pain from an infected tooth being pulled. I look down at my ankle, and see it is now a dark color and very swollen. The pungent smell of old, stale sweat fills the room. There is a severe pressure sore—black, damaged tissue encompassed by angry red and inflamed skin sullies my once healthy leg. Everyone notices, but no one says a word. Mom quietly covers her nose, horrified.

"What happened?" she asks quietly.

"Whoever put this cast on applied it too tightly. This is compartment syndrome," Dr. Aston explains. "Very, very painful," he says, shaking his head.

He pats my leg gently and continues to shake his head. "We'll take care of this. No more cast," he assures me as he loosely applies a padded ankle splint.

"Just be careful, no quick movements, and keep an eye on that ankle for the next few days. You can apply a light moisturizer cream and increase pain medication. Let me know if anything worsens."

"Thanks, Doc," Dad says as he helps me off the exam table back into my wheelchair.

Dr. Aston stoops down and pulls me into a fatherly hug. "You've been through so much, Cait, especially for someone so young," he says softly.

"Thank you," I manage weakly through my exhaustion. I've been battling the pain for so long, but also recognize this feeling of relief at having that cast off.

The second we get home, even before I'm transitioned out of my wheelchair back into bed, Mom applies a generous amount of coconut oil to the pressure sore on my ankle.

"What are you doing, Mom?" I ask her curiously as I watch her dip her fingers into a jar of semi-solid white stuff and wipe it over the black sores on my leg.

"I've heard coconut oil is a cure-all, so let's just see what happens," she replies, wiping the greasy substance onto a paper towel.

"I guess it can't hurt," I agree and am secretly glad to have the smell of earthy coconut take over the smell of decaying flesh.

*   *   *

I sleep most of the day. Even the smallest outings drain my body of energy. Dad comes into my room to check on me late that afternoon.

"How about that wheelchair ride now?" he asks me in his typically good-natured way.

"I look a mess. I don't want anyone to see me like this," I answer, staring down at my unshaven legs peeking out from the bottom of my purple nightgown.

"You look fine. I bet no one is even outside. Come on. You need to get out of this room." He is already at my bedside, ready to lift me out and into my wheelchair.

"Alright. Fine. Let's go," I agree begrudgingly.

Dad rolls me through the house, out the front door, and down the ramp until we are outside in the bright Florida sun. I hear a little whimper—my little fox-like dog, who has started joining us on these outings, doesn't want to be left behind. Dad scoops him up and sets him on the pillow in my lap.

I'm glad to be outside again. The sun on my face and the fresh air always ease my pain and anxiety.

"Cait, I want to talk to you about something," Dad starts hesitantly.

I know where this is going.

"If it's about the lawsuit, I don't want to go there," I respond sharply, cutting him off before he even starts.

"We're coming up on the six-month mark of your accident, and you're still in bad shape. We don't know what the future holds for you, physically. Your medical expenses are well over a million dollars by now, and thank God, Mom and I have great health insurance. I just feel you should be compensated for something like this."

The word lawsuit floats around in my mind, heavy and unrelenting. It's not just about the energy it would take—energy I don't have right now. It's about what it would mean. Pursuing a lawsuit feels like admitting defeat, like accepting the label *permanently disabled*. And I am not permanently disabled. I won't let that be my truth. I refuse to surrender to it. Not here, not in my lifetime. That's not who I am, and it never will be.

"No. I don't want to do it," I reply flatly.

Dad sighs, and I can sense his frustration. I know he means well.

"I wish everyone would quit telling me they don't know what the future holds. I'm going to get better, Dad. I'm young and I'm strong. I can't live like this forever, and I won't give up until I get back to being *me* again."

"I know. We just want to make sure you are taken care of, that's all," he answers quietly, pushing my wheelchair further down the sidewalk.

We don't say much for the rest of the ride. Dad wheels me back into my room, and my body is aching relentlessly from sitting up straight for too long. He lifts me from the wheelchair and helps me back into bed. I hate this hospital bed, but I'm also grateful for it. It has become a security blanket of sorts, the only place where I can find even a semblance of comfort.

I look around my room. There's not much to do besides read or watch TV. Those tongue depressors are still staring me in the face. It has taken longer than anticipated to pry my mouth open, but I'm finally able to enjoy solid foods again. It's brought a new joy into my life; I get excited about food like I never have before, carefully planning out my menu each week. Papa, my grandfather, stops by most days of the week with a Whataburger or some delicious treat in hand and my mouth salivates whenever I consider what my next meal could be.

This is quite the change for someone who was living off protein shakes, "healthy" Lean Cuisines, and obsessively counting calories in college. As I consider whether to ask for a bacon cheeseburger or Subway for dinner, I realize that none of that matters anymore. Even if they weren't the healthiest options, they were nourishing me in a way that fed my soul, and that's exactly what I needed right now. For the next few weeks, I happily devour bags of salt and vinegar potato chips, mint-flavored Oreos, chocolate milkshakes from our local Tastee Freez, and cheeseburgers from Whataburger.

I set down an empty glass of milk next to my half-eaten box of mint Oreos on my bedside food tray. Even though all this food has brought a glimmer of joy back into my life, it hits me that I'm still stuck. Nothing has really changed other than I can eat again, and while I'm grateful for that, I can't just lie in this bed forever and eat my life away.

I turn my focus to my right leg, still wrapped in a soft-fitted cast. The coconut oil has helped heal the pressure sore and the skin over my ankle looks almost back to normal. *It really is versatile*, I think about the oil.

I stare at my toes and try so hard to wiggle them. Nothing. No movement.

Okay. Maybe just my big toe. I concentrate even harder. *Just move. Come on. MOVE.* Nothing.

Of course there's no movement, what did I expect? My sciatic nerve was severed.

I quickly turn my head to the side, trying to hide my tears and frustration. It's been almost six months. I was sure the nerves would have started to "wake up" by now. I place my fingers on the outside of my right thigh, which feels more like a large bone from all the muscle wasting away. I start scratching the outside of my leg and notice feeling in my toes. I scratch harder and feel an intense burning and tingling in the tips of my toes as I continue scratching. There's still some sensation, but it doesn't feel like my leg anymore—it's as if someone has superglued this random leg to my body.

I hear footsteps coming down the hall and stop at my door. "Cait, we are leaving in twenty minutes for your appointment," my mom calls out.

"Okay!" I yell back. Today I'm going to be fitted for an ankle foot orthotic, or AFO. My surgeon explained it's a device designed to keep my foot, ankle, and leg from dragging on the ground once I'm weight-bearing.

It's a forty-minute drive to the Hanger Clinic. Mom and I are silent for most of it. As we pull into the parking lot, I get a sinking feeling in my gut.

"I don't want to go."

"Why? This is a good thing, Cait. It's one step closer to you becoming more mobile," mom tries to assure me.

"I don't know. It just feels too permanent—like the paralysis will never get better if this is what we do next."

My mom sighs heavily as she opens the car door and prepares to get out. "Don't look at it that way. There's still a small chance the nerves will regenerate. Do you remember what the doctor said?"

"Yeah . . . I know . . . give it time . . . but it's been six months." I hate how my voice has an edge of whining to it.

"Let's just go inside, let them look at your leg, and see what recommendations they make."

I don't look up, just nod my head. A part of me feels embarrassed and ashamed. This kind of thing doesn't happen to someone like me—I'm young and athletic. Or at least, I used to be. I grit my teeth, fighting back the urge to cry.

Just suck it up. Get a grip, Caitlin, I scold myself.

Mom wheels me into the office, and we are immediately called back. A nice woman walks in, carrying what looks like several leg braces, and places them on a counter.

"Okay, let's get you fitted. I know these can look scary and complicated, but they will make a big difference as you become more mobile and keep you from tripping over your own foot."

"That's great," I reply with a forced effort and feigned excitement.

Brace after brace is applied until we find "the one." I stare down in horror. *I have to wear this big, bulky robotic contraption?* I feel gratitude for the brace and its capabilities and anger and frustration over my situation and the robot monster I have been turned into.

I need to get out of here. I sigh heavily and lay back on the exam table.

Mom sees I am growing weary and tries to hurry the process along.

As we check out, mom hands the orthotic brace to me and I place it over my lap. We then make our way to the car. The second the car door shuts, I burst into sobs. I can't hold back the tears any longer.

Mom doesn't say anything. She just places her hand on my back to comfort me. I lean back into the seat as I wipe tears from my eyes.

"My body burns and aches all over, Mom," I whisper in defeat.

She quickly reaches inside her black leather purse and pulls out an orange pill bottle. I hear the familiar click of the white cap as she unscrews the lid. I grab the white circular-shaped pills from her and pop them into my mouth.

The pain nearly steals my breath away. It feels as if someone has relentlessly whipped the lower half of my body with a leather belt, until it's raw and inflamed, exposed. That's nerve pain for you. Comfort becomes a distant memory. I've come to realize that while the pain medication offers some relief, the intense discomfort never truly leaves me. It's a relentless, unending torment, hovering just beneath the surface of my reality, always threatening to break through. Every twinge, every sharp pang, is a reminder of Dave and the hell he put me through. Anger bubbles up inside me, a hot, bitter wave that crashes over my thoughts. *How could he be so careless? How could he ruin my life and walk away unscathed?* Some days, I wish he could trade places with me, just for one day. I imagine him trying to go about his normal routine with this chronic pain, so intense it completely debilitates you and makes even the simplest tasks feel insurmountable. The more I dwell on it, the angrier I become. I picture him, carefree and oblivious, and it makes my blood boil. This bitterness is a poison, seeping into every part of my being. I know I can't stay in this place too long or it will swallow me whole, but sometimes it's hard to escape the haunting memories of that day and the life I lost.

*   *   *

Though pain is still present, I continue to progress in physical therapy. After six months in a hospital bed, every single muscle in my body seems to have forgotten its purpose. My doctor says it is time to start pool therapy—that the water will support me in ways the harsh, unyielding ground can't. The buoyancy will allow me to stretch and strengthen muscles that have atrophied during my months of immobility. Pat is my therapist for the day, always vibrant and full of energy. I alternate between him and another therapist for my three-day-a-week sessions.

"What have you got there with you today?" Pat asks as my mom wheels me into the clinic.

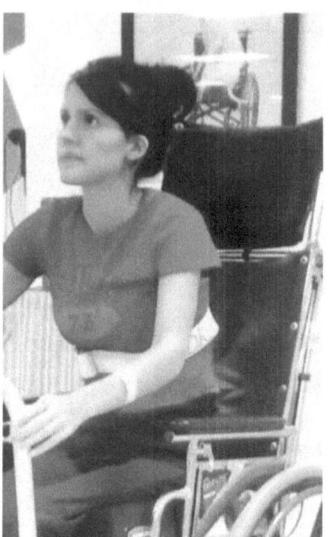

I look down at my brace and shrug. "It's my new orthotic," I answer, trying to hide my disappointment. The brace has become not only a constant reminder of the accident and its impact on my mobility, but it's also uncomfortable and cumbersome.

"Well, have you named him yet?" Pat asks jokingly, picking it up off my lap to get a better look.

"Nope. He won't be hanging around long, so he shall remain nameless," I say with a smile. Pat nods and smiles awkwardly. "Well, you ready to get started?" he asks.

I nod enthusiastically. "My brain says it's ready, but I don't know about my body."

We make our way to the women's locker room, and Mom helps me change into a swimsuit—a two-piece tank top and shorts, such a stark contrast from the Quicksilver bikinis I used to wear on the beach, another sober reminder of how much my life and body has changed.

"All set?" Mom asks, wheeling me around to face the mirror.

I immediately roll my eyes when I notice her laughing.

"I guess this is what it took to finally get you into one of my 'old lady' suits," she jokes.

"Very funny, Mom," I laugh. The sound startles me—laughter, something I haven't done in six months. For so long, my days have been a blur of pain and therapy. But this moment, this simple act of laughing, feels like a return to something normal and familiar.

Mom wheels me into the pool therapy room. *How the heck am I going to get into that pool?* I wonder. *I can't just walk down the steps.*

Pat enters the room through a side door. He has a walker in his hand and places it in front of the pool lift chair.

Sudden understanding dawns on me. *Oh, that's how.*

"Okay—Mom, I want you to wheel Cait over to the chair, and I'm going to help her stand. Cait, I want you to try to balance on your left leg while holding onto the walker, and then we'll ease you into the chair." Pat hands out instructions like a pro.

I immediately tense up because I know more pain is coming. Mom wheels me to the pool chair, and Pat firmly places his hands under my armpits as he lifts me out of the wheelchair and positions me in front of the walker. My left foot comes in contact with the hard surface of the floor, and I try to steady myself.

"I've got you," Pat says assuredly. "I won't let go," he promises.

I place my hands in a death grip on either side of the walker and stand upright for the first time in months.

"I want you to carefully hop to the pool chair using just your left leg. I'm right behind you."

I survey the distance between where I am "standing" to the where he wants me to go and think it is an impossibility.

I try to hop, but my body just won't move. It feels so unnatural, and I'm scared I'll shatter my bones or bust one of the screws holding my pelvis together. The pool chair is just a couple of feet in front of me but feels like it might as well be a few miles.

I can do this.

"Trust me," Pat says. "You're going to be fine."

I carefully and slowly hop my way to the pool chair, Pat holding onto my back the entire time. It is really more of a shuffle than a hop, but I decide I don't care, because I am moving on my own.

Pat then helps me into the chair. For the first time, I look around and notice other therapy patients in the water. They're all much older than me, probably in their late seventies or early eighties. I feel like I don't belong here and am hit with a wave of sadness.

"You okay?" Pat asks, noticing my shift in energy immediately.

"I'm good," I answer, trying to hold it together.

Pat nods and explains he is going to press a button that will automatically lower me into the pool. "I'll be down the steps in a flash to meet you."

I nod my head to indicate I understand and brace myself for the feeling of the cold water washing over my body.

Pat presses the button, and the chair swivels to the side and begins to lower me down. Sure enough, Pat is there to meet me. And then something strange happens—the pain is gone. I feel nothing—no discomfort, nothing. It's like I'm floating on a cloud. I start smiling and can't stop.

"It feels good, doesn't it?" Pat asks, noting the smile on my face.

"It sure does," I say, surprised. Pat places a float in front of me, and I grab hold of it as I ease myself off the pool chair.

"Today, you're just floating. No walking. I want your joints to get used to movement again, and I don't want to push it to the point where you're in a lot of pain after therapy."

I nod, too focused on the sensation of my body moving and the absence of pain to respond. I surprise myself and actually choke up as Pat slowly glides me through the water. It feels like heaven. I don't want it to end. We drift to the deep end, and I let go completely, relaxing my body.

We make our way back to the shallow end of the pool and I strike up a conversation with a group therapy class. They have so many questions for me. "What happened?" "How long is your recovery?"—they genuinely seem interested in my case.

"You're so young to be going through something like this," one of the ladies blurts out.

"Yeah, I guess I am," I nod.

As we continue to discuss our various injuries and ailments, a realization dawns on me—there are so many people experiencing pain and suffering. It's a humbling thought to see how widespread and varied our struggles are. My own story seems to resonate with them, breaking the stereotype that pain is something only the elderly endure.

Determined to connect with others on a deeper level, I decide to make a conscious effort to get to know my fellow patients and learn about their healing journeys. I jot down their names and stories in my journal. Each week, I meet more people—young and old, from all walks of life. There's a sense of camaraderie that begins to form, making my therapy sessions something to look forward to. Not only because it is the only time where I am free from pain, but it's the time where I can connect with someone and something outside of my pain.

As the warm water cradles my injured limbs, I take my first "steps" in the pool. The therapy group gathers around and cheers me on. Placing one foot in front of the other, I wobble and sway, like a toddler learning to walk for the first time. Pat supports me, steadying my faltering steps. I manage to make it to the wall and back twice before needing to take a rest. For the first time since this ordeal began, it feels like I'm truly making strides forward—I can see and feel real progress!

After pool therapy, my mom helps me dry off and change into clothes; Pat hooks me up to an electrical stimulation machine hoping to elicit some movement in my leg and foot.

As I lay there, praying for movement, I ask Pat if I can come in five days a week for therapy, instead of three.

Pat pulls up my chart and answers, "Well, your doctor requested only three days of therapy, and to be honest, you probably need some downtime to recover from all the work you have been doing here. But I tell you what, the doors are open anytime you and your mom or dad want to come. You're always welcome."

I nod as I stare at my motionless leg and foot. "Thanks, Pat. I need to put in more hours. Push harder, ya know?"

He nods in understanding but cautions me gently, "We don't want to push too hard and have setbacks. You're doing way more than we had anticipated. Be proud of yourself and take it slow."

I don't do slow, I answer him in my head as I paste a fake smile of understanding on my face.

* * *

Mom and I are silent on the ride home from therapy. The aftermath of each session is brutal—my pain levels skyrocket for hours after exerting so much effort. Nights are especially rough, leaving me with little chance of sleep. I hesitate to increase my pain medication because it turns me into a zombie the next day, so I ask for ice packs instead. Dad brings me a couple, and I methodically rotate them from my jaw, neck, shoulders, back, tailbone, and across my pelvis. Ice and water therapy are the only things that provide any relief.

As I will myself to sleep, I think of a story Pat had told me about one of his past patients, a man in his fifties who had survived a horrible motorcycle accident and had severely shattered his pelvis, just like me. He had also found immense relief when submerged in water, so much so that he installed a hot tub on his front porch and practically lived in it. A nurse checked in on him periodically, and he had people delivering his meals, which he ate while soaking in the tub. His neighbors thought he was just lazy until they learned about the accident. As I reach for another ice pack and apply it to my neck, I can't get that man off my mind. Once I'm allowed to take baths again, I've decided I'm going to live in my bathtub.

Another week of pool therapy goes by, following the now familiar routine: walking in the water, floating for pain relief, a few hops on my walker, then electrical stimulation. Swimming is strictly off-limits because too much movement could cause serious harm. I must be cautious, restricting myself to small, controlled movements in the water. While I'm submerged, the pain subsides, but I've learned not to push it. The pain always comes later, like a delayed reaction—or punishment for wanting to get better.

"Time to do some floating," Pat announces, handing me an oversized red foam noodle. I grasp it and let my body go limp, eyes closing as I surrender to the moment. Then, for some reason, I open my eyes and glance to my left; I notice someone who looks a lot like Dave seated in a chair, watching me.

It is *Dave!* I realize and nearly fall off my float. *When did he slip in?* I wonder angrily.

My body tenses immediately.

"Everything okay?" Pat asks, noticing my hard-earned moment of zen has been replaced by something even I can't define.

"Yeah, it's just fine," I respond, locking eyes with Dave. He gives me a head nod before continuing his chat with my mom. I try to ignore his presence, the critical gaze I feel on me. Pat helps guide me to the pool chair and meets me at the top with a towel and my walker.

"I'll let you get dried off and changed, then meet you in the therapy room for some electrical stim," Pat explains.

I nod, as Pat wheels me up to the locker room, my mom trailing behind. "Mom, did you know he was coming?" I hiss in a frustrated whisper.

"No clue!" she replies, wheeling me into the changing room.

"He just loves being mysterious and showing up unannounced," I say flatly.

"I wish he would at least give us a call or text," Mom agrees.

It makes my blood boil. I am seething.

We make our way to the main therapy room, where Pat is ready and waiting with all the equipment set up. He helps me onto the padded table, attaching various wires to my legs before turning on the machine. It's slightly uncomfortable but not painful—finally.

Dave sits quietly in the background. We have barely acknowledged one another. He then pulls out a video camera and starts filming me. I don't say anything to avoid a scene, but the atmosphere grows awkward. After a few minutes, he puts the camera away.

Dave gets up to help me into my wheelchair, but Pat beats him to it, sensing my discomfort and taking his role as my therapist to the next level, as my protector.

"Okay! I think that's all for today," Pat announces, flipping the wheelchair's leg supports around and expertly placing my feet on them.

"Thanks, Pat. See you next week." I make eye contact with him, trying to communicate what I can't say out loud.

Mom pushes me down the hall with Dave close behind. "I need to use the restroom. I won't be long," she says, as we exchange glances.

Dave and I are finally alone. I study his face. It's tense, every line etched with anger. "I can tell you don't want me here," he spats out finally.

"How can you tell?" I reply sarcastically, shifting my tense body in my wheelchair. Mentally screaming at him for coming and ruining my few moments of relief.

"I can't believe they call this therapy," Dave scoffs, pulling out his phone to review the video he had taken without my consent.

"What?" I ask incredulously, genuinely puzzled by his sudden outburst.

"I'm not impressed with what I saw today. You just floated in a pool and laid on a table. They should have you on ellipticals or stationary bikes. Maybe you should find another rehab clinic. This one is a joke." His eyes narrow as he continues to point out the weaknesses of the clinic.

"So, what facility would you recommend for injuries like mine?" I snap. "I'm sure your graphic design degree makes you more knowledgeable than my trauma surgeon, you know, with his fifteen years of education, and all. You have no idea what I've done to get here. You only see snippets of my life. You have no right to judge." I pause, my breathing heavy. Making a decision to draw a line in the sand that I know I will never cross over again.

"Leave, Dave, and this time don't come back. Ever."

Dave laughs, smugly. "I know you don't mean that." His look is challenging and full of self-pride.

"No. I mean it," I answer emphatically, anger and resentment filling my throat, forcing the words that I have so needed to say since the day this happened, out of my heart and into his face.

"I don't want to ever see you again."

Unbeknownst to me, Pat was nearby catching up on some paperwork and overhearing our conversation. He walked up just as Mom exited the bathroom.

"Maybe you should just leave," Pat says sternly to Dave. Motioning with his hand the direction Dave should take to go.

Dave glares at Pat for a few seconds and turns and leaves without a word.

"I'm sorry," I sob to Pat.

"Who is that jerk anyway?" Pat asks, compassion filling his face as he comes over and stoops down to my level.

"He's nobody," I answer, wiping tears from my eyes.

Pat nods sympathetically, patting my shoulder. "He sure is," he says in agreement.

Mom and I make it to the parking lot just as Dave's car speeds off, tires screeching as he peels away in anger. Throughout the day, he bombards me with text messages of old photos of traveling or at the beach, even sending me a picture of a cute puppy he found on the side of the road—anything to tug at my heartstrings. I can tell he's panicking. He senses a change in me. A strength that has never been there before. I delete them all without hesitation, feeling a weight lift off my shoulders as I erase him from my life.

I hope he stays away . . . for good this time.

* * *

Today, we're heading to Mobile, Alabama, for my appointment with Dr. Carter, my orthopedic trauma surgeon, who had been hand-picked by Dr. Anderson, my surgeon in Dallas. Dad and Mom pack a cooler with food and plenty of ice packs.

Throughout the car ride, I rotate the ice packs on and off, shifting uncomfortably in my seat. Sitting in an upright position continues to be one of my greatest struggles. I try not to focus on my pain. Instead, I think through my appointment and concerns I want to discuss with Dr. Carter.

"Hello, Cait! How's my girl doing?" Dr. Carter greets me with his warm, familiar smile and strong Hispanic accent as he steps into the exam room.

I reply that I'm fine, but we both know it's a lie.

"You say the same thing every time we meet, Cait. I know you are not 'fine,'" he calls me out without hesitation. "Give it to me straight."

"Honestly?" I hesitate for a minute but decide that if I can't be honest with my surgeon, who can I be honest with? "I'm frustrated," I admit, my voice cracking. "I'm not progressing fast enough in therapy. I want to start running and working out again.

I'm tired of lying around all day. And the pain—I can't take it anymore. It feels like this will never end." I begin to cry and bury my face in my hands.

"How much longer do I have to live like this? Can you give me a date? Anything? Can't you tell me how long it's going to be before I'm better?" I know he can't, but I plead anyway because I have reached a level of desperation I didn't know exists.

"Her boyfriend came into town and told her he wasn't impressed with her progress," Mom chimes in, feeling the need to give some context to my breakdown.

"Mom!" I snap, embarrassed by the truth.

Dr. Carter sighs, his expression softening with empathy. He turns in his revolving lab stool and grabs a Styrofoam cup from the countertop, then positions his chair in front of me.

"See this cup?" he asks.

I nod, puzzled, wiping my face with my shirt.

In one swift motion, he crushes the cup with both hands. I jump at the swift motion, but am brought back around to the sober reality of my situation when he says simply, "This is what happened to your body." He pauses to let his message sink in, and then moves on.

"Caitlin, the active girl you once were is no more. I'm sorry," he continues, his voice gentle yet firm. "I am honest with my patients because I don't want to give you false hope. Your injuries were very severe. I am so impressed with your strong will and determination. I know you are used to the 'no pain, no gain' mentality, but this is not that—it will not work for this. The more you push, the greater the pain and setbacks. You need to come to terms with the fact that your body is now very fragile, like that of an elderly woman."

I nod, fighting back more hot tears.

"Dr. Carter," I finally speak up when the most intense emotions have moved through me. "I appreciate your honesty. I really do. But that's not going to be me. I just can't accept that. I may have some limitations for life, but I won't be permanently disabled. I *will* get back to being active again. My cousin's wedding is next summer, and I plan to be out on the dance floor with my family."

Dr. Carter smiles, a sad yet hopeful smile. "I really do hope so!"

We continue with the exam.

On the ride home, I try not to dwell on Dr. Carter's words, but the crushing sound of the Styrofoam cup keeps ringing in my ears. As fear and anxiety creep in, I breathe it out. It's hard to hear these things about my body, my life, but I know, if I am going to get better, I can't accept them as my truth. I won't. Ever. I am tired of so much, but mostly, I realize, I am exhausted from all the talking about *me* and my injuries. I'm not broken. At least not permanently.

As the car moves down the highway, I close my eyes and make a silent promise to myself. No more doubts, no more letting others define my limits. I will overcome this. I am not broken.

I am not broken.

TWELVE

FROZEN PEAS

I lay back on the padded table, its meager support doing little to ease the constant ache in my tailbone. It makes me think about how it was crushed upon impact with the hard pavement. The squishy ball in my hand, given to me by Dr. Bennet's nurse, is already under the tight grip of my fingers. I brace myself for the inevitable pain as sticky pads are placed all over my legs, feet, and ankles; the cold sensation of each one is a prelude to what's coming next.

Click. Click. Click.

The sounds of the EMG—electromyography—machine hum in the background; the only glimpse I caught of it was when my grandfather and I first entered the clinic's back room. Dr. Bennet sits to my left, methodically opening small packs of more sticky pads. The crinkling noise fills the sterile room as I lift my head from the small pillow and see an array of needles, some small, some alarmingly large, being prepared. Wires dangle from them, ready to connect to the machine. I tense up, forcing myself to look away and lie back down. The waiting is the worst part, knowing pain is just around the corner. Sweat beads on my forehead, though the procedure hasn't even started. My unshaven legs and bare feet burn with a dull, persistent pain. My stomach growls, reminding me of the breakfast sandwich I couldn't bring myself to eat due to my anticipatory anxiety.

"I'm going to turn on the machine now and we'll get started. Just hold very still and let me know if you need a break," Dr. Bennet says, his voice steady and calm. As a longtime family friend, Dr. Bennet has always demonstrated an exceptional bedside manner unmatched by any other doctor I've encountered. If I have to endure this kind of pain, I'm grateful it's him by my side.

I had been warned that grown men have cried out during this procedure, some unable to make it through to the end. The lightest touch or a sheet brushing against my leg sends a shooting pain through my body on even the best of days. *How am I supposed to endure needles being inserted into these hypersensitive areas?* I wonder as I stare up at the ceiling. Once the needles are placed on my right foot, the doctor activates the machine, sending electrical shocks into my body to stimulate the nerves. For someone with severe nerve damage, it can be excruciating.

"Okay. Here we go," Dr. Bennet informs me. I nod, close my eyes, and take a deep breath, trying to relax my body.

Don't look. Don't look at the needles. I urge myself to find something pleasant to focus on.

Dr. Bennet gently grips the bottom of my right foot. "Take a deep breath," he says, "I'm going to start at the bottom and work my way up."

Oh, great. I wish he didn't need to start at one of the most sensitive areas on my body.

I feel the needle pierce the bottom of my foot, and a scream escapes my lips as pain radiates up my right leg. My body is drenched in sweat. The red squishy ball in my hand feels like it's about to burst from my grip.

"I'm sorry," the doctor says, with genuine sympathy in his voice.

Another needle is inserted, then another. I grit my teeth, my body trembling with the pain. My grandfather rises from his chair, his eyes locking with mine, filled with the desperate desire to pull me out of this nightmare. He paces for a moment before sitting back down.

"Do you need a break?" the doctor asks.

"No. Keep going." I force the words out, knowing this test is crucial. It measures the nerve and muscle activity to assess the damage and see if there's any regeneration. My need to know how I am progressing outweighs my physical discomfort.

More needles. More pain. Larger needles this time, gripping the edge of the exam table as I register feeling the thick tacks piercing my skin. I picture myself in the medieval times, laid out on a torture table, shocked over and over again. Panic rises in my chest, my throat tightens, my face flushes. My ears ring, and everything fades to black.

"She's passing out!" my grandfather's voice breaks through the haze as I hear his frustration and panic.

The machine is turned off. I feel my grandfather's hands helping me sit up on the table. The doctor returns with a cold water bottle, pressing it against my cheek. As I start to come to, their voices echo around me.

"Are you okay, Cait?" The doctor asks, with genuine concern. "I think that's enough for today," he says as I struggle to make my eyes focus. "You are one tough cookie,"

"I feel like I'm going to vomit!" I cough and try to hold back last night's dinner as the trash can is brought over; I hunch and vomit up the contents in my stomach. My grandfather hands me paper towels, his eyes glistening with tears.

"I know that was very painful. We got a partial reading, but we'll need follow-ups every six months to track your progress," the doctor explains.

I don't respond; just hang my head in defeat.

"I'm so sorry," my grandfather whispers as he and my grandmother help me into the car, where she had been waiting.

"I won't be doing a follow-up," I declare, a sob taking hold of my throat. "That was torture. I don't care to know how much nerve activity I have anymore. It's not worth it." I sag into the back seat of the car and let the tears fall.

"It's a shame you have to go through all of this, Caitie," my grandfather says, using the nickname he's called me since I was a child. "All because of that idiot." He climbs into the driver's seat and slams the door shut a little too hard, for emphasis.

The rest of the drive is silent. I know the "idiot" he refers to—Dave. My family never liked him, and even more so now after the accident.

Back at home, I lie in my hospital bed, tears streaming down my face. The events of the day have left me shaken, trapped, and overwhelmed by a paralyzing fear. It's not just fear of the unknown, but a deep-seated fear of my body. The pain. *What if this is as good as it gets?* I wonder, a chilling realization grips my heart. I keep getting knocked down, time and time again. In my mind, I envision a giant hammer pounding me into the ground, relentless and unforgiving, pounding me into a state of nothing.

As I sink back into my hospital bed, it dawns on me. Part of the heaviness I've been carrying is grief. It's been quietly settling in, perhaps for longer than I care to admit. Retrieving my laptop from the nightstand, I type into the search bar: "The stages of grief." As I read through what pops up, "Denial, anger, bargaining, depression, acceptance." I feel a resonance followed by the swift gratitude that denial, at least, has long since slipped away from me.

My emotions swing wildly between sadness and anger as I mourn the girl I once was. Even with friends and family around, I feel deeply alone. Isolation, pain, and a sense of losing myself consume me. The urge to hit the pavement and run until I can't is overwhelming. Running used to be my escape, my way to numb my emotions. Whenever life became too much, I'd lace up my shoes and run until I felt nothing. It was my drug, my coping mechanism.

But now, running isn't an option. My body won't let me escape that way anymore. The pain demands to be faced head on—because the alternative means I will be crushed under its weight.

I reach for an old Bible, a gift from my grandparents for my sixteenth birthday. It had spent most of its time tucked away on a shelf, gathering dust next to a stack of nonfiction books and fitness magazines. But now, it stays on my nightstand, close at hand. I often read from Psalms, finding comfort in its verses framed around happiness, peace, and contentment. Tonight, I turn its pages aimlessly, reading snippets here and there without fully comprehending. Then I stumble upon the book of Job.

I immerse myself in Job's story, my eyes blurring with tears as I read and reread his journey of questioning and seeking. Like Job, I grapple with the incomprehensibility of my own suffering. Yearning for clarity, I wonder, *Could there be a greater, divine purpose unfolding beyond my understanding?*

In the quiet of my room, I ponder my path forward. One certainty emerges amid the uncertainty: I have to keep moving forward. My gaze falls on the turquoise notebook, used for documenting my journey post-accident, tracking medications, and jotting down thoughts. Flipping to a blank page, I pen in bold letters: "My broken body does not mean I am a broken person."

With deliberate strokes, I sketch out charts outlining personal goals, marking achievable milestones and setting aside space for progress notes, inspirational quotes—anything to motivate me along the way. In my mind, each goal, from standing with my walker for five minutes to using light weights for arm exercises in my wheelchair, was a step toward reclaiming my quality of life. Among them, "Finish College Degree" stood alone on a separate page.

Pausing to contemplate, I pick up my laptop and navigate to the college application page. The upcoming fall semester is only a month away. Three classes seem daunting, considering all the pain I am in while sitting in an upright position. With a racing heart, I complete the form and hit send.

Here goes nothing.

Closing my laptop, I adjusted the incline of my hospital bed. Out of the corner of my eye, I notice my four-legged mobility aid with its sturdy frame of steel positioned next to my nightstand. I was given this walker at the pain clinic to help with my limited mobility. I don't care for it much, but I have no choice if I ever want to walk again. Bracing myself, I roll to the side and struggle to push myself up with my arms, my muscles protesting with each movement. My pelvis and its construction of screws, chains, and titanium plates, radiates pain with every effort.

Ignoring caution, I grasp the walker and slowly stand. I smile mischievously knowing my parents will absolutely disapprove of my attempt at doing this on my own. I hesitate, feeling the weight shift awkwardly, but determination spurs me forward. One tentative hop, then another and another—each movement cautiously planned out in my mind. With gritted teeth, I make my way to the door, navigating the pain that pulses through the lower half of my body with small stops and rests.

In the living room, my mom's startled gaze meets mine, her coffee almost spilling out all over herself when she sees me enter the room. For a moment, I feel like a child caught in an act of rebellion, yet beneath her surprise, I sense a glimmer of pride.

"What are you doing, Cait?" Mom asks frantically, hopping up from her chair, looking for a safe place for her coffee cup to land.

"Oh, you know—just testing out my capabilities. I can't lie in that bed forever. Plus, I need a timer."

"Well, I could have gotten that for you," she says, a twinge of frustration in her voice as she just stands there, staring at me helplessly.

"I know," I reply nonchalantly. "So, do you have a timer I can use?"

"Yes, but let me help you back to bed and then I'll bring it to you. You're crazy, ya know? Dr. Carter said not to use the walker without assistance."

I roll my eyes and offer a closed-lip smile.

"Look, I want you to progress, but you must be careful. You also have surgery in two weeks to remove the IVC filter. Take it easy."

Thanks for the reminder.

I had forgotten about the IVC filter. It was placed several months ago near my heart to prevent any blood clots that could result from my lack of mobility.

"Look, I promise I won't try anything unless I am 100 percent certain I can do it safely."

"I've heard that one before," Mom jokes, leaving the room in search of that timer.

"Remember the time you 'safely' climbed up a sixty-foot cliff and jumped into the water because someone dared you to do it? I don't have to remind you about the whiplash you suffered and blurred vision that followed as a result, do I?" she called over her shoulder.

"Got it, Mom." I know she means well.

I hobble to bed, and Mom follows to lift my legs around into position. I feel my body give out as I sink into the mattress. For the rest of the day, I time myself standing on and off, using the walker for support. I decided not to push it too much; just that little hobble to the living room caused me significant pain. I write down notes on today's progress, feeling a small sense of accomplishment.

My brother is expected to arrive shortly and will stay with us for a while. He just finished his baseball career at Florida State University, which ended with a severe shoulder injury. *We should be two peas in a pod,* I think. I am looking forward to having him here to break up the monotony.

Mom makes a big dinner that night for my brother's arrival, and we all gather around the table. I use my walker and slowly hop to the table. There's a donut-shaped cushion on the seat of the wooden chair and a soft pillow for back support. This is my first time sitting in a chair in six months. Dad carefully helps me into the chair and scoots me up to the table. This is also the first time I've seen my brother since the accident.

"I can't believe everything you have gone through," my brother says as he stares at the girl I've become. I can tell he is looking for the real "me" wondering if she is in there somewhere.

"It hasn't been easy," I respond, carefully navigating a spoonful of pot roast into my mouth. Even though I've managed to stretch out the space between my jaws, there is still a significant amount of pain if I stretch too far to eat.

We all dig in, and for a moment, the conversation pauses as we focus on enjoying our meal.

"Well, I did something today!" I blurt out.

Mom and Dad exchange glances and then look in my direction. I know they are holding their breath.

"I'm going back to college in the fall," I announce happily, an assured smile fixed on my face.

"What?" Mom asks, completely stunned.

"Yep, I'm not waiting around any longer. I'm getting on with my life." I ask my brother to put some more potatoes on my plate and look at my dad for his endorsement.

"But Cait, your doctor discouraged this. Please just wait another year. You have already had so much stress on your body." My mom hasn't touched a thing on her plate. She pushes the food around with her fork, but it never gets anywhere near her mouth.

My brother gets in on the conversation and cracks an all too familiar joke. "Mom, there's no use in trying to reason with her. Cait's gonna do what she wants to do. You know that!"

My dad clears his throat and takes a sip of water. "If she feels like she can do it, then we need to support her." He is resolute in his statement.

"You know we will," my sister chimes in, raising her eyebrows at my mom.

Realizing she is outnumbered, my mom gives in. "Of course you will have our support."

"Well, it's settled then. I start in a month."

Ten minutes pass and dinner is nearly finished when the pain in my tailbone and back become so unbearable that I can no longer focus. I can't sit anymore. I'm in too much pain. I need my wheelchair.

"I'll make it work," I reply with an assurance that comes from deep within me. Closing my eyes, I take a deep breath and blow through the pain.

Dad pushes me back to bed. Mom brings the rest of my dinner on a tray and hands it to me, but I am no longer hungry.

My brother, concerned, follows with a confused look on his face. "I didn't realize it was this bad, Cait. You can't even sit in a chair for more than a few minutes."

I looked up at him, exhausted, I didn't feel like explaining everything to him and simply said, "I can, but I have to be medicated. I just need another dose of painkillers."

He picked up the orange bottles of pills lining my bedside table and read the names of the medications out loud. With raised eyebrows he didn't say what I knew he was thinking: This is some strong stuff. Instead, he placed them back in their neat rows and asked, "How long will you have to be on these?"

I shrug as I wipe sweat off my face with the top bedsheet. All the exertion of trying to attend dinner out of my bed had caused me to break a sweat.

"My doctor says I may never get off them. I don't know," I shrug.

The look on his face is one of pity. I hate being pitied.

"I hate seeing you like this," he murmurs gently. And as if an afterthought, he looks me right in the eyes and states, "And I really hope you get rid of Dave."

I looked out the window as I contemplated how to answer.

"I don't know where we stand right now, but I did tell him never to come back here again."

He shook his head in disbelief that I could still be in communication with this guy who almost ended my life. But then all of a sudden it was like he understood that I was just trying to survive, and that Dave was the least of my problems. He patted my leg, the right one that had no feeling, and said, "That's at least a start," before walking out of my room.

Another week crawls by and I come to a decision. I am getting out of my hospital bed today. I make this declaration to my mom when she comes in to administer my pain meds.

"I want to sleep in a regular bed. I don't want to be tethered to this hospital bed any longer."

"Are you sure you're ready? A regular bed won't have the water insert," she cautions. The water insert was prescribed to help prevent bed sores and make the nerve pain more bearable.

"I'm sure," I reply, gripping my walker as if it was the last line between me and a life of dependency. "And I need to start showering by myself, going to the toilet alone, making my own food. I want my independence back." I watch my mom closely for her reaction. I know I am going to meet resistance, but I also know I need to reclaim a little part of my independence if I am going to survive the next phase of my recovery. If I don't take these small steps toward independence, I'll be at risk of relying on someone's help forever, and that is something I could not, would not, allow to happen. Before the accident, I was fiercely independent. Even as a toddler, I'd look my mom in the eye and declare, "Me do it!" As much as I appreciate the support and care from my family, it is time for me to start pushing myself. Healing isn't just about physical recovery; it is about reclaiming my spirit, about fighting to be the person I was before the accident, and about making sure I stay on the right path.

"You have never been one to take things slow, have you?" My mom eyes me as she folds a basket of towels at the foot of my hospital bed. She grows quiet, almost thoughtful, as she gathers the folded fabrics to put them in their place in the closet at the end of the hall. She concedes with a sigh, "If you feel ready, then go for it." And then she walked out the door.

I am ready. My heart knows I am ready, even if my body hasn't gotten the message yet.

With Mom's help, I transfer to my wheelchair, and she and Dad set to work dismantling the hospital bed to make room for the standard full-size bed frame and mattress that have been sitting in storage. Mom calls the medical supply company to arrange the pickup of my hospital bed. As they set up the new one, I can't help but smile thinking about how good it will feel to sleep in a regular bed because it will be the most normal thing I've done in six months.

"It's all set up!" Dad announces proudly.

Mom hands me my walker, and I hobble to the edge of the new bed. With their help, I ease myself onto the mattress. But as I settle in with just one pillow, I quickly realize it's not going to work—the strain on my pelvis is too much. Seeing my discomfort, Mom leaves the room and returns with an armful of pillows, placing one under my knees and arranging five more to prop me up.

"This is going to take some getting used to," I admit, trying to find a comfortable position.

"I told you this is too soon," Mom says, with a tinge of frustration in her voice and raised eyebrows.

"Maybe so, but I'm still glad I did it," I retort through gritted teeth.

Six months. I spent half a year of my life in that hospital bed. And now, I'm done. I've had enough. I know my body isn't quite ready, but I don't care. I can't stay in that bed a minute longer. Even if it means more pain, I need to feel like I'm moving forward, like I'm not just wasting away. Transitioning to a regular bed—it's a small thing, something so ordinary that most people wouldn't even think twice about it. But for me, it's monumental. It's the first real taste of normalcy I've had in what feels like forever. I need to feel like I am taking control, like I am returning to some semblance of a life that feels like mine.

I can't sleep at all that night; the pressure on my joints from the mattress becomes unbearable. The nerve pain feels like hot sores have opened up all over my body. Reaching for my cell phone, I dial my parents' home number. Mom answers, her voice groggy with sleep. "I need ice packs," I say quietly, begging for relief.

"Okay, I'll get them," she responds, still half asleep.

Mom walks into my room, arms loaded with several bags of frozen green peas. The doctor wasn't exaggerating when he recommended them; they work better than any other ice pack I've tried, despite their small size. She hands them to me one by one, and I place them on various parts of my body. The ice-cold packs make me tense up, but I know from experience that I'd rather be cold than in pain. I finally doze off, shivering under my blanket, the faint smell of frozen peas lingering in the air.

I wake up the next morning to the unmistakable odor of thawed peas. I shift slightly to the right, pulling my sheet closer, and my hand brushes against a pile of tiny cold balls. I freeze, my brain slowly catching up with what's happening. Peas. One of the bags must have popped open during the night. Slightly annoyed, I start brushing them off the sheets with quick, irritated swipes, like I'm trying to erase the mess from existence.

When I had first returned home, word of my struggle with pain and sleepless nights spread throughout our community. Soft pillows, bottles of Biofreeze, and other thoughtful items began appearing on our doorstep. The gift that stands out the most is a homemade ice pack, meticulously sewn together by a kind friend. It is brightly colored, filled with what feels like patches of rice, and large enough to cover the entire lower half of my body.

That first time, as I placed the ice pack on my body, I mar-velled at the care and effort that went into making it. *How lucky am I? Someone cared enough about me to thoughtfully construct this.* The ice-cold sensation sent shivers through me, but I hardly noticed because I knew relief was coming. Pulling my thick comforter up to my chin, I laid still, letting the icy pack work its magic. The flames of pain coursing through my body gradually subsided, and I finally relaxed.

*　　*　　*

Over the past few weeks, I've noticed the oxycodone is becoming less effective. My pain management doctor suggests increasing the dosage, but I'm reluctant. I know these medications aren't good for me in the long run, and I dream of a day when I won't need them anymore. Determined, I pull out my journal and write "Goal: Get off all painkillers."

It's not going to be easy, and I don't know when or how it'll happen, but I refuse to rely on these pills forever. The thought of being free from medication is enough to fuel my resolve. If I have to permanently attach ice packs to my body to numb the pain, so be it. I envision myself using an Ace bandage to wrap cold compresses around my limbs; anything to escape the cycle of medication.

I'm further motivated to get off the painkillers because I'm noticing their side effects are outweighing their benefits. The crippling fatigue they leave me with feels permanent, never mind the severe constipation those meds treat me to—bottles of orange-flavored MiraLAX have become a staple for me to help with bowel movements. My stomach aches and hurts after every meal, and I can't tolerate even a few sips of coffee without experiencing burning pain in my abdomen.

And a quick Google search about other symptoms that plague me confirms my suspicions: The painkillers are causing my headaches, nausea, blurred vision, and confusion. Not to mention that words are starting to slip away from me. Just the other day, I wanted to ask Mom for the remote but couldn't find the word. I knew what it was in my head, but I couldn't make the word come out of my mouth. It scared me.

I decide to check my school inbox and see an email about one of my upcoming college classes. *How will I get through college if I can't even remember what to call a remote?* I wonder.

*　　*　　*

My first day of school arrives sooner than expected. My sister and I sit shoulder to shoulder in the backseat of my grandparents' Honda; they have generously volunteered to get me to classes so my parents can get back to work. In the back of my mind, I hear the voices of my parents, as well as my surgeon, telling me to wait, that it's too soon. The parking lot seems enormous, far bigger than I remember, and the sheer magnitude of crossing it amplifies my anxiety. My heart races, pounding against my ribcage like a trapped bird.

Maybe it is too soon. I start to shake and sweat with realization that I might have bitten off way more than I can chew right now.

The thought of navigating the bustling hallways and keeping up with the pace of school life suddenly terrifies me. It hits me that I have a real fear of my own body now. The constant, nagging pain and discomfort, along with the bouts of severe pain that strike without warning, make me feel like a stranger in my skin.

I turn to my sister and grandparents, contemplating asking them to turn the car around, to take me back home. My mouth opens to speak, but the words catch in my throat.

I want to get out of here. My mind is screaming, but I can't find the words to say it.

Up until this point, I have barely left the house, with the only exception being for therapy and doctors' appointments. As we sit here in the parking lot, in the back of my grandparents' Honda, the minutes stretch on. The comforting scent of my grandfather's peppermint gum mingles with the faint smell of the car's interior, grounding me slightly. I can feel my sister's eyes on me. With a deep breath, I try to muster the courage to move forward. The car door handle feels cool, and I grip it tightly, still torn between staying and going.

"You alright?" my sister checks in.

"Yeah, just nervous." I look over at her, willing myself not to cry.

"You don't have to do this," she tells me, as she puts a reassuring hand on my arm.

"No. I need to do this. If I don't, I'll never move forward." I take a huge deep breath and gather all my courage and strength. It is now or later, and I am so tired of living for later. I need things to happen *now*.

My sister helps me out of the car and sets my black donut cushion onto my new, smaller wheelchair, which is easier for me to navigate. Balancing on one leg and holding onto the car for support, I carefully lower myself into the seat.

"You got this, Cait," my sister whispers into my ear, reassuring me as she hands me a notepad.

"We are just a phone call away, please call if you need us." My grandmother leans down to plant a warm kiss on my cheek.

I put my sunglasses on to hide the fear in my eyes.

"Thanks! I'll be fine," I respond, though my voice carries more apprehension than confidence. I hope desperately that they don't notice.

I watch their white car pull out of the parking lot and realize, for the first time in over six months, I'm on my own. If this is what anxiety feels like, then I've got it.

I wheel myself up to the sidewalk, stopping to take in my surroundings. Everything feels different. I'm different. I see students walking with excitement, I can feel it in the air—it's the first day, the start of a new school year. But I don't feel excited.

I look toward the building where my class is and notice a young girl in a wheelchair. She seems happy and content as she sips her drink and basks in the warm sun, face upturned, soaking it all up. A deep sadness comes over me, not for my situation but because I realize I probably never would have noticed her before my accident. I was too busy socializing, hurrying to class or hitting the gym to pay attention.

Suddenly, I recall my five-year-old self seeing the elegant woman in a wheelchair at the restaurant my family often visited. I shyly handed her a crisp five-dollar bill, my young, compassionate heart thinking maybe she could use it. Her long, blonde hair cascaded over her shoulders, and her radiant smile met mine as she accepted the gift. In that moment, I saw how she navigated life with grace despite her limitations. Her resilience was a silent yet powerful message to me: If she could find joy and continue forward, so could I.

I hesitate slightly, but before I know it, I find myself rolling my wheelchair toward the girl sitting nearby in her own chair. She greets me with a warm smile, and as we start talking, I learn that she was born without the use of her legs—this is the only life she has ever known. Instantly, we connect. Our conversation flows naturally, as we share our stories, hopes, and fears without a trace of judgment. It strikes me how rare it is to form such a genuine connection, free from any superficiality. We chat a bit longer, exchange numbers, and go our separate ways.

I wheel myself down the hall, careful not to hit anyone with my chair. When I enter the small room filled with at least fifty computers, I'm greeted by the professor. "Hello!" I say, trying to mask the fear and anxiety coursing through me. He genuinely smiles and asks if I'd like a seat up front to accommodate my chair better.

I shift uncomfortably on and off through class, pain is my constant companion whether I am in class or in bed. The professor dismissed us early, and I dial my sister's number to pick me up.

"Well, how was it?" she asks, eager to hear about my day.

"Different. It's all so different. I'm just glad to have the first day behind me. I am having trouble focusing in class though. The pain is so bad, and I can barely stay awake. Probably from the pain meds." I feel like I'm about to drift off, just talking about it.

"Maybe you should talk to your doctor," she suggests.

"Yep. I'm going to."

The moment I arrive home, I call the nurse at my pain management doctor's office. By evening, I have a prescription for Adderall in my hand. I've heard of it but never tried it—it's supposed to help with focus in class. My doctor also mentioned it could help with my pain.

I decide to tuck a small bottle away in my purse, for emergencies—like those moments when I can feel myself nodding off during lectures.

The next day is quiet and mundane; I don't have any classes. I spend it practicing with my walker, navigating the familiar spaces of my home, from my bed to the bathroom, then to the end table and the dining room table; I make the rounds repeatedly. My fingerprints leave smudges on everything I touch, a tangible record of my progress. I try out my dad's recliner and can tolerate it well. Mom brings me a large pillow under my knees for support and another for under my right ankle. I stare at my ankle, which dangles to the left side of the pillow, and focus hard on my toes, trying to get some movement. Then something strange happens. It feels like a bolt of electricity going through my leg and into my big toe—and to my absolute shock, it moves! Just a little flick to the right, but it moves!

"It moved! It moved!" I scream.

"What moved?" Mom, startled by my reaction, runs into the living room worried about the scene she might encounter.

"My big toe! It moved!" I look at her for confirmation.

"You're kidding!" she exclaims, examining my foot skeptically.

"No, I'm not. Watch!" I focus hard, and again, my big toe shifts slightly to the right.

"Oh my gosh! Cait! This is great news!" Mom exclaims excitedly. I can't help but smile.

"I'm going to be on the dance floor next summer at Blakely's wedding and I'm going to hike the Grand Canyon from rim to rim with Dawna!" I promise. Watching to see if my toe will move again.

Mom's face shifts from elation to sadness as she tries to share in my joy.

"You don't think I'll be able to do it, do you?" I ask her, an edge of disappointment in my voice. There is a part of me that doesn't understand why my own mother can't believe in me the way I do.

"I'm just going off what the doctor has said, Cait. We need to be realistic. I don't want you to get your hopes up."

"Mom, there was movement in my toe, and that's all the motivation I need!" I'm defiant and definite. I will walk again.

Mom offers a faint smile just as my stomach lets out a loud gurgle.

"What's for dinner tonight?" I ask, changing the subject.

"Chicken, potatoes, and . . . peas," my mom replies with a laugh.

"No, not my peas!" I chuckle but am also kind of grossed out at the thought of eating my "ice packs" for dinner.

"Don't worry, your grandfather brought you an entire cooler full. You should be good for the next few months," she reassures me as she moves back into the kitchen to finish the dinner preparations.

After dinner, I hobble to bed using my walker, each step deliberate and slow. I carefully lower myself onto the mattress where Mom is ready to help lift my legs. I sink into a mountain of pillows that cradle my aching body. Reaching for my water bottle, I take two oxycodone from the nightstand and swallow them down, hoping for relief. Mom places the small red and white cooler next to my bed; it's packed with frozen peas for when the pain inevitably wakes me in the middle of the night. As I think about the slight movement felt in my toe earlier, a flicker of happiness sparks within me—an emotion that has been absent for so long. I immediately reach for my journal and write under the progress notes "Movement in big toe!" I can't help but smile, a real genuine smile, as I close the journal and set it aside. Finally, I drift off to sleep, the smell of frozen peas filling the air, and for the first time, I feel a glimmer of hope, the size of a small green frozen pea.

THIRTEEN

NOTHING LEFT
TO BREAK

I stare down at the bulky brace, strapped tightly around my right leg. My brother jokes that it looks like something ripped straight from a sci-fi flick—cold, metal, robotic. The brace is supposed to keep my lifeless leg, ankle, and foot from dragging behind me. No matter how much I beg my body to respond, the paralysis won't give an inch. All I can manage is a pathetic twitch of my big toe. What was once a flicker of hope has become a cruel reminder of everything I can't do. It's like my own body is taunting me, dangling the possibility of movement just out of reach, only to snatch it away again.

The heat is unbearable as Florida's relentless humidity wraps itself around me, making the padded brace stick even more to my sweaty skin. My calf feels like it's suffocating under the pressure of the device. I shift uncomfortably in the passenger seat of my sister's car, wishing she would hurry up. I pull out my phone, hoping for a distraction and the date slaps me in the face. April 21. It's been over a year since the accident. A year. *How is that even possible?*

Progress has been excruciatingly slow, a crawl that feels more like trying to dig my way out of quicksand. I'm moving, but barely, and I'm not getting anywhere. Most days, I'm trapped in a loop, like living the same day over and over again. Bed to recliner, recliner to the back porch, back porch to the shower, shower back to bed, rinse and repeat. Physical therapy and school are the only things that break up the monotony, but even those sometimes feel like a cruel joke. I go to class once a week, but have to do the rest online because I can't physically sit through an entire day in a classroom without popping pain meds like they're candy. At least at home, I can lie in bed with my computer, ice packs numbing the pain. "Two years." The doctor's words hang in the air, heavy and ominous, like a curse that's been placed on my life. Two years before I might—just might—feel a little less pain, before I can move a little more freely. "We don't have a crystal ball," he added. "There's no way of knowing what you'll be left with."

Two years. That's also when I'm supposed to taper off the max doses of prescription ibuprofen. The anti-inflammatories are nonnegotiable right now, crucial to keeping the swelling down around my pelvis and backside where the soft-tissue damage is still a raging inferno inside me. But with every pill I swallow, my stomach issues get worse. I can feel it. It's like trading one agony for another. And yet, I have no choice but to keep popping these pills.

"Took you long enough! I'm dying in here," I snap, my irritation bubbling to the surface. The heat is suffocating, causing the sweat to pool under the brace, which is driving me crazy.

"Sorry! I couldn't find the keys," she says. "Plus, Mom had a million questions for me."

I crank the air conditioning up to full blast, letting the cool air wash over me as I sink back into the black donut cushion in the passenger seat. My sister's been taking me out once or twice a week for little outings. Most of the time it's just to a store in town; we don't do much besides walk the aisles, but it's the closest thing to normal I can manage. At least it gives me a chance to practice walking with my walker, to see if I'm getting any better.

The blue handicap sign swings back and forth from the rearview mirror as she hits a bump in the road.

"I hate that thing, you know?" I mutter, watching it sway.

"Well, I love it!" Ash jokes, trying to lighten the mood. "I get all the good parking spots thanks to you!"

"Glad I could help you out there," I reply, a half-hearted attempt at humor.

"Where do you want to go today?" she asks, changing the subject strategically.

"We could try Publix, I guess. I need some coffee anyway." The words come out of my mouth like they are nothing. I want to sound casual, like this is just another errand on just another day, but the truth is, it isn't. Just getting myself ready in the morning—holding my arms up to brush and blow dry my hair, struggling through the simple act of dressing—sends pain shooting through me, sharp and relentless. The kind of pain that would bring anyone else to their knees, but for me, it's just the start of the day.

We drive in silence, making our way through the parking lot's maze. I scan for a spot that isn't marked with that blue and white sign, the one that screams "You don't belong here!" every time I see it.

"I don't want to park in a handicap spot if we don't have to."

"Okay, but you know you're allowed to, right?" my sister peruses the long line of cars parked in the lot, looking for a close enough spot.

"Yes, I know, but I'm not handicapped!" The words come out sharper than I intend, laced with anger I can't control.

"Whatever you say," she mumbles, rolling her eyes.

I glare at the handicap tag swinging from the mirror, feeling the shame bubble up inside me. It's ridiculous, I know. But there's a part of me that wants to rip it down, chuck it out the window, and pretend for just a moment that I don't need it. If I can't see it, maybe it won't be real.

We circle the lot again, my eyes scanning for an open spot. Not a single one up front . . . except for the dreaded handicap spot. Of course.

Ash pulls into it with a grin, ignoring my silent protest. I can't help but laugh, despite myself, shaking my head as she hops out of the car. Before I can even brace myself, she's already got the walker out of the backseat, ready for me.

"I don't want to use the walker today. Just put it back," I bark my order, hauling my already weary body from the car.

Ash looks from the walker, to me, and then back down at the walker again.

"What? Cait, you have to."

"No, I don't. Just put it away." I am already making progress toward the front door of the grocery story. I'm unsteady, but my irritation at being labeled handicap is keeping me propped up as I drag my braced leg behind me.

"Why are you doing this to me? Why not wait for Mom to test out your capabilities? What if something happens?"

"I'll be fine. Plus, you'll be there to catch me, right?" I force a smile, trying to mask the mix of determination and fear. Ash helps steady me on my feet, her hands gripping mine tightly. I had walked through the house without the walker before, but I always had a wall or furniture to grab onto. This is different. It was just me and the open air, and a whole lot of concrete.

"You can let go. I'll be fine," I say, trying to inject some confidence into my voice, even though I'm not sure even I believe it. I start inching toward the store, and with every step, I make a careful negotiation with the ground beneath me. My fingers skim the cold metal rails lined with shopping carts. The concrete feels unpredictable under my feet, every crack and bump a potential threat. I scan the path ahead, hoping my body will cooperate long enough to get me inside.

Out of nowhere, a voice cuts through the quiet; a man's yell echoes across the parking lot. I pause, looking around.

"Is he talking to us?" I ask my sister, confused.

"I don't know," Ash responds, her eyes narrowing as we both turn to look. The man is moving closer, his voice growing louder and more agitated.

"You know that's a handicapped spot you girls are parked in? That's a $200 fine!" he shouts in our faces, his words sharp and accusatory.

Ash and I freeze, the reality of what's happening taking a moment to sink in. The man keeps yelling, his voice grating on my nerves, pushing me closer to my mental edge. My heart races as I realize he has no idea. He can't see it—the brace under my pants, the paralysis, the chronic pain. I guess I look normal. Normal. That word feels like a joke.

We turn away from him, our faces burning with embarrassment. But he keeps coming toward us. I lean on Ash for support, the anger boiling inside me, my Southern manners wearing thin.

We reach the double doors of the store, and I stop, unable to hold it in any longer. "Cait, just keep going. Don't say anything. I don't want to cause a scene," Ash whispers, pleading.

"He's already caused a scene," I say loudly, spinning around to face him, my eyes locking onto his.

"Sir, my time is limited, and you've just wasted five minutes of it," I snap, the words tumble out before I can stop them, frustration seeping into every syllable. "So do us all a favor—shut your mouth and quit following us." The anger in my voice surprises even me, but I'm too far gone by this point to care.

The man steps back, his face pale, silent for the first time. I hold his gaze, daring him to say something else. Ash tugs at me, urging me to move on, but my heart is pounding, adrenaline surging through me.

We continue into the store, and then we hear it again. "I see you got a little limp!" he yells, his voice dripping with sarcasm, insinuating I am making it up.

People are staring now; there is a crowd of eyes on us.

"How embarrassing!" Ash mutters, shaking her head.

"The nerve of him!" I spit out, the anger still simmering.

I cling to the shopping cart as we move through the store, every step sending jolts of pain through my body. But there's something comforting about being here, out in the world, even if it's just a grocery store where we are being chased by the world's rudest customer. It feels almost normal.

We make a loop around the store, Ash grabbing a bag of Columbian coffee and a few additional items for Mom while I find a wooden bench to rest on. The pain radiates in my back, neck, and shoulders, muscles spasming and tightening relentlessly as I try to find a comfortable position to rest. The nerve pain shoots from my pelvis into my feet as I shift uncomfortably. I know I'm running out of time.

Ash wheels the cart over, and I slowly stand, using it to steady myself. My right leg now feels like dead weight, as I drag it behind me. We head toward the exit, both scanning the parking lot, wary of that man showing up again. The sight of our car brings relief. For once, I'm actually grateful for that blue sticker.

We weave through the lunch traffic in silence, both lost in our own thoughts. I never know what kind of day I'll have when I wake up. Some days are "good pain days," but even those can knock me flat. I wonder if this is my new normal, if this pain is here to stay. I do my best to push those thoughts down, but my mind is restless.

I can't stop thinking about that man in the parking lot, and then my thoughts jump to the week before, to that awkward moment in a restaurant with my family, when we bumped into some of my parents' old friends. They asked what I was doing with my life, and their question landed like a punch to my gut. I felt a flash of fury—how dare they? My instinct was to scream, "I'm just surviving over here!" But then, the realization hit even harder—no one could see the reality beneath my skin. They couldn't see the bones, held together by screws, bars, chains, and bits of titanium— all things that don't belong in a human body. They couldn't see, let alone comprehend, what it felt like to have severe and permanent nerve damage that burns through me like fire.

They weren't there to witness the white, circular-shaped pills I had swallowed so that I could just look presentable, or sit upright, so that I could suffer in silence through the agony of just existing at that moment. The frog-in-a-blender analogy my surgeon used, brutal as it was, rang so true; it was almost deafening.

I despise the way I feel the need to validate my existence to others—to justify my pain, my struggle. Like the random guy in the pain management waiting room who told me he had a hip replacement and now he's walking around just fine, with no pain. "You're young and you'll be running around in no time!" he said, so cheerfully. My jaw tightened as I felt the sharp sting of those words.

We pull into the driveway. My mom is already at the door, her face a mix of concern and determination as she moves to help me inside. As soon as I'm through the door, I head straight to my bed, the only place that offers any semblance of relief. Collapsing onto the mattress, I feel the weight of the day settle into my bones. My mom stands nearby, propping pillows under my right leg, now swollen and an angry shade of purple. The lack of blood flow makes it look more like it belongs to a corpse than to a twenty-four-year-old woman. But I've learned to ignore it—just another part of the new normal.

I lay there, staring at the ceiling, my mind drifting to the future. In a week, I'm supposed to graduate from college. I also have a surgery scheduled the day before to remove the IVC filter that's been sitting near my heart, warding off blood clots. I'm more mobile now, so my doctor said it's finally safe to remove it. I should be excited about graduation, about walking across the stage and grabbing the diploma I worked so hard for. But all I can think about is the pain—the inevitable pain that comes if I push myself too far. As much as I want to be there, to feel that moment, I know deep down it's not worth what my body will have to endure.

"Mom, I'm not sure I want to go to graduation next week. There'll be a large crowd, and I don't want to dope myself up just to get through it," I say, breaking the silence. My voice sounds hollow, even to me.

"Are you sure? It's a big deal that you graduated. You might regret not going one day," my mom replies, studying me skeptically.

"I know how many painkillers it would take to make it through that ceremony, Mom. It's not worth how bad I'd feel afterward."

She nods, her eyes softening in the way they do when she knows I'm right but wishes things were different. "I get it," she says softly.

*   *   *

The surgery to remove the IVC filter is over before I can even process it, a whirlwind of hospital lights, sterile smells, and the sharp sting of needles. I'm in the car, heading back to Florida from Dallas, the miles rolling by like the blur of the last twenty-four hours. My arms bear the proof of it all, a patchwork of black and blue bruises from where they tried, and failed, to find a vein. In the end, the nurse had to go for the one in my left foot, the last resort before they could put me under.

I lean my head against the car window, closing my eyes as the sun's warmth seeps through the glass, a rare comfort amidst everything else. The thought crosses my mind—*by the end of today, I'll be a college graduate.*

But then what? What comes next?

One day at a time.

It's all I can manage right now. If I think too far ahead, panic creeps in, a slow, insidious weight pressing on my chest. My cousin's wedding is in a few weeks in Orange Beach, Alabama—the same place where I met Dave. Just the thought of going there makes my stomach churn. So much time has passed since then, and yet, here I am, stuck in this place of loss, while time marches on, indifferent. It's a cruel thing, how time and loss dance around each other, never quite in sync. Time doesn't care. It doesn't slow down or wait for you to catch up. But loss—loss stays. It digs in, dragging grief, pain, memories—all of it—along for the ride, refusing to fit neatly into the world's timeline.

I realize I'm on the outside now, disconnected from the life I once knew. It's like I've been yanked out of that river in North Carolina my family used to frequent, left to stand on the shore, dripping and cold, while everyone else floats by, oblivious. Loss is lonely that way. It sets you apart, makes you different. I know I can't go back to who I was before. I've changed. My wants, my dreams, my desires—they're all different now. Once your health is gone, everything else seems so small, so insignificant. The world keeps turning, but I'm standing still, trying to make sense of it all.

The day of my cousin's wedding arrives like a freight train, I've been bracing myself for the impact. I sit in the corner at the reception, my bright blue silk bridesmaid dress spilling over the sides of my wheelchair; I'm doing my best to look as if I belong there. The pain has clawed its way through the layers of painkillers I've taken just to make it this far, and I'm barely holding myself up. My mom is off to the side, talking to the chef about making an ice pack for me in the kitchen, her eyes full of the same worry they've carried since the accident.

Michael Jackson's "Thriller" starts to blare through the speakers, and instinctively, everyone rushes to the dance floor. It's the kind of song that usually pulls me up and out too. I can almost see the version of myself I thought I'd be tonight, laughing and spinning with the others, the pain, a distant memory. But here I am, watching from the sidelines, feeling more defeated than I've ever admitted. The sadness and grief sit heavy in my chest, threatening to break me down right here in front of everyone. I lean over to my mom when she returns, "I can't do this anymore," I say quietly. "I want to leave."

We say our quiet goodbyes; I'm trying to mask the devastation in my voice. My mom wheels me out to the parking lot, and as we approach the car, a black Audi parked next to it catches my eye. Dave. He's been texting me intermittently since last time at pool therapy. I've only responded enough to update him on my progress. He knew I'd be here tonight; his parents' condo is within walking distance of the venue. But I wasn't expecting him to actually show up.

He steps out of the car, and my mom looks at me with wide eyes, the unspoken question clear: Did you plan this? I shake my head slightly.

"What are you doing here?" I ask, my voice flat, weary from pain and another disappointment.

"I just want a minute of your time, that's all," he says, his hands going up in front of him, as if he is trying to say, "I surrender."

I slump down into my wheelchair, the energy drained from my body.

"It won't take long," he insists.

"No," I say quietly as I look up at him.

"No?" he repeats, surprised, like it's a word he's not used to hearing.

"No," I say again, more firmly this time. "Mom, let's get in the car."

Without another word, my mom helps me into the passenger seat, while Dave stands there, awkward and unsure. As we drive away, it doesn't take five minutes before my mom spots his Audi in the rearview mirror.

"He's behind us!" she says, with a mixture of disbelief and fear.

"Don't pull over. Just keep going," I tell her.

"You don't think he'll do anything crazy, do you?" she asks, the fear evident in her eyes as she takes her gaze off the road to check in on me. We exchange glances, both knowing that we can't really answer that question. "Cait, maybe it's time to move on . . . for real this time," she says gently.

"I know," I respond, glancing at the car behind us. My phone vibrates with another text from him, but I ignore it.

Mom veers into the right lane, and Dave follows suit, staying close behind us for the entire forty-minute drive to my grandparents' condo where the rest of our family is staying for the wedding. We pull in, and Dave pulls in right behind us.

"I can't believe he has the guts to just follow us like that. I'm calling your dad," my mom says, her voice shaky with exhaustion.

"No," I respond calmly. "Help me out of the car and then leave us. I'm ending this, once and for all."

Mom looks at me, clearly not wanting to leave me alone with him. I know she'll be calling my dad the second she's out of sight, rallying the troops.

She hands me the walker just as Dave steps out of his black Audi. The crunch of gravel under his leather sandals grates against my nerves, each step bringing him closer. Mom doesn't take her eyes off him, her gaze hard and unflinching, as if daring him to make a wrong move.

The salty air clings to my skin, mingling with the sticky residue of the evening; I lean against the car, my fingers gripping the cool metal of my walker. My blue bridesmaid dress, now marked with the wear of the night and dotted with stains, drags along the asphalt, collecting dirt. I inch forward, the familiar weight of my body shifting onto my well-defined arms, now the only part of my body that is strong from months of dependence on this metal frame.

Dave stands a few feet away, his arms crossed, eyes narrowed with that infuriating smirk playing on his lips. It was a look I had grown used to, the one he wore whenever he thought he had the upper hand. I can tell he is trying to read me, trying to find a crack in the mask I've carefully put in place, looking for any sign of weakness.

I don't hesitate. The words spill out as if I've rehearsed this moment countless times in my mind. "I'm done. It's over, Dave," my voice is steady, unwavering. My message is clear.

He scoffs, his mockery, which used to pierce me deeply, barely registers. "I've heard that before. You think you can just walk away from this? From me?"

"Yes. I can, and I already have." I have never been more resolute.

There's a moment of silence between us. I can tell he knows I am for real this time.

Dave crosses his arms, his smirk widening. "You've had months to try and get better. I gave you time and space," he pauses. "And just what are you going to do with your life? Who's going to want you like this?" He gestures dismissively at my walker, his smirk shifting to disgust.

I don't flinch. I just stare at him, letting his words hang in the air, absorbing their sting and letting it dissipate into nothingness. There was a time when they would have torn me apart, but not anymore. Not after everything I've already endured.

"I will be okay. I will get through this. But you . . . you will have to live with the fact that you nearly destroyed a life for the rest of your life."

He tries to interject but I cut him off with a raised hand.

"You can't hurt me anymore, Dave." My tone was matter of fact, as though I were stating a simple truth. "You've done everything you could do. There's nothing left to break."

I brace for his comeback, but it doesn't come. He's silent, fully aware there's nothing left for him to say or do. He's lost all control. I can see him struggling for a response, but he's at a loss.

"Goodbye, Dave," I say softly, forcing him to meet my gaze one last time. The words catch in my throat, heavy with their finality. He stands there in the driveway, motionless, as if he's still waiting for something—for me to say more, to take it all back. I turn away from him as I shuffle through the condo parking lot, the clatter of my walker echoing harshly against the cold pavement. The sound bounces around me, starkly contrasting to the waves' soft, rhythmic crashing in the distance.

I don't look back. But I can feel his eyes on me, a burning weight between my shoulder blades. Part of me wonders why he stayed so long. Was it guilt? A twisted sense of obligation? I don't have the answers, and it doesn't matter anymore. None of it matters anymore.

In this moment, I start to release everything I've been holding onto—the shouting, the belittling, the relentless chipping away of who I was. I see his hands around my neck, the force with which he threw me. I see myself flying through the air, glass shattering around me like deadly confetti, the world spinning and then—impact. The sickening crunch of bones against asphalt, the searing pain that erupted and swallowed me whole. I see the girl who lay crumpled on that road, broken in every way possible, her spirit shattered just as thoroughly as her body. I let go of the endless wondering, the gnawing worry of what really caused the accident that night. I'll never know.

I picture all that suffering, physical and emotional, gathered up and cast into that same ocean I swam in hundreds of times since I was a kid. I imagine it being carried away, absorbed by the vastness of the sea. In the end, the waves take it all, leaving me with a strange sense of release, a quiet space where I can finally begin to heal.

FOURTEEN

BUTTER KNIFE

I'm sitting on the couch, legs stretched out, propped up on the coffee table. The pillows tucked beneath them feel like they're holding me together. Another firm cushion supports my back. I'm staring out the window of my grandparents' condo, watching the waves of the Gulf crash against the shoreline, doing everything I can to ignore the knot twisting in my stomach. Any minute now, a knock on the door will come. A part of me still doesn't get why they're coming at all. *I mean, they want me to sue them?* It sounds absurd, and once again I feel like I am playing out the plotline of some weird drama. *I'm not even disabled. I'll be back to myself in no time, right?*

I rock my aching body from one side to the other and catch my breath in pain. *Who am I kidding? I can barely sit up for twenty minutes without relying on a cocktail of painkillers to numb every-thing.*

Mom is in the chair in front of me, her nose buried in a book, while dad is in the kitchen preparing spaghetti for dinner. I watch him move around with that constant energy of his, like he's chasing some rhythm only he can hear. We call him the Energizer Bunny because he never stops. I got that from him, and it's killing me now, not being able to move the way I want. It's a quiet kind of torment, being a restless soul trapped in a broken body. Hearing the rhythm but essentially too paralyzed to chase it.

The knock comes and it feels like the whole room freezes. My dad stops stirring the pasta, my mom nearly drops her book in her lap. We were all expecting this visit, so I don't know why we were all surprised that they are actually here now. We all glance at the door, like what's on the other side of it is going to reveal some big truth we aren't ready for. Dad's the one who moves first, heading over to let them in. I shift, wincing, trying to sit up straighter. I even did my hair today, and I had made the extra effort to put on some makeup. It cost me an extra pain pill but holding the blow dryer and brushing on some blush felt like a worthy price for a little bit of dignity.

"Hello," a voice says as soon as my dad opens the door. It's all too familiar and too distant all at once. Dave's dad. I haven't seen him in over a year, not since I was residing, or rather surviving, in the trauma ICU unit. I was in so much pain I barely registered who he was through the haze of morphine.

Everything about this feels wrong.

Does he know Dave and I aren't together anymore? I wonder as I watch him walk into the living room.

Before I can find the words to break the awkwardness, Susan—Dave's mom—sits down next to me, pulling me into one of those warm hugs of hers. "You look so great! How are you doing?" she asks, her soft Southern drawl conveying real interest.

I smile and lie through my teeth. "I'm doing fine." Susan's always had this way of making people feel like they matter, like you're the most important person in the room. Even now, after all we had been through, I still felt it. Then Richard speaks, cutting through our connection. "So, you were able to finish college?" he starts. No preamble. Just straight into it.

"Yes. Even though my surgeon advised me not to. He thought it'd be too much stress on my body."

"And how was it?" The question sounds innocent enough, but I know where this is going.

"It's been tough," I admit. "Managing school while dealing with the chronic pain and relying heavily on painkillers was challenging, but I'm relieved to have made it through."

He nods, but I can tell it's just a prelude. Before I know it, the interrogation starts. Questions rapid fire at me, each one chipping away at whatever composure I thought I had come into this meeting with. His tone is gentle, but something feels off. Richard has always been kind, even before the accident but today he's different—more probing, almost interrogative. It unsettles me, though I can't quite place why. *Is he concerned that I might sue him personally, instead of the insurance company?* The thought lingers, leaving me feeling uncomfortable. It's a stark contrast to the Richard I once knew.

The questions continue.

"How much pain are you in right now? On a scale of one to ten?" I half expect him to pull a notebook out of his shirt pocket and start documenting my answers.

"Do you have days without pain?" he goes on.

"How are you getting around?" He looks around the room, apparently looking for evidence that I am able bodied and just blowing this whole thing out of proportion.

"Have you considered getting a job?" Sweat beads on my skin as the truth slams into me with brutal clarity: He doesn't believe me. Or maybe he does, but this is just another layer of protocol, legal jargon he's been told to dish out to people like me. People who are broken but look whole. I don't know. What I do know is without the wheelchair or the walker chained to me twenty-four seven, I must look fine. Maybe even normal.

The mascara clings to my lashes, thick and dark, making my eyes look brighter than they are. A soft sweep of peach blush brings life to my cheeks, and slick of lip gloss gives my lips a shine that almost feels real. It's all a mask, though, painted on to hide the fractures underneath—both physical scars and emotional wreckage. The layers of makeup are a barrier between me and the truth—how broken I really am.

They don't see the scars tucked inside my mouth or the story carved into my bones. The left side of my jaw split in half, snapped like brittle glass in the crash now held together with metal bars and tiny chains, pieces of me tethered back in place like I'm some twisted sculpture. The right side? That was obliterated too—bones shattered into pieces. The doctors didn't want to ruin the right side of my face, so they went in through my head, pulling my skin and muscles aside like curtains to fix what they could. And that's just the top half. The lower half of my body is a whole other battlefield of hidden wounds.

And if anyone looked at me now, sitting on this couch, pretending I'm fine, they'd never know. They wouldn't see the truth—the pathetic truth of how broken I am. How I've become an expert at faking it, at hiding pain.

I zone out for a second, catching my breath. He keeps pushing on with his questions.

"I heard you went to your cousin's wedding. How was that?"

I pause and fire back, "I wanted to be there but it didn't go how I anticipated." My pain meds are wearing off, and I can feel that familiar ache returning to my lower back.

"Oh? Why?" his eyes narrow as he continues to inspect me—mentally taking notes of what is seemingly *not* wrong with me.

"I was in so much pain that I had to leave the reception early," I explain. I wait, as he stares at me expectantly. *Okay, I'll give him more.*

"Sitting, standing, walking—it just gets worse with every movement. It's like my body is one giant, raw open wound. The only thing that helps even a little bit, is lying down with ice packs placed all over my body and painkillers. I spend my days planning for and around my pain." I stop and take in his face, along with

Susan's. Her eyes have filled with tears, and her mouth is trembling. His eyes, on the other hand, are completely devoid of emotion.

"I don't know how I'm supposed to live the rest of my life this way . . ." I trail off and grimace, moving my right leg from the pillow that is keeping it propped up.

"I see." His tone is clinical, like he's just checking boxes; once again, I'm an object to be studied and reported on.

"Has the paralysis gotten better?" he asks, staring at my leg.

"I can move my big toe, but that's it," I respond flatly.

"Can I see?" This time, his question seems to feel inappropriate, even to him, but he pushes through.

I hesitate but agree. "I guess so."

Awkward doesn't even begin to describe how I feel as I reach under my thigh, lifting my leg so he can watch the pitiful movement in my foot. I can feel my parents' eyes burning into us, their discomfort palpable. Susan shoots her husband a look that screams *What are you doing?!*—but it rolls off him like he doesn't notice or care.

"Try moving your ankle," he says.

"I can't!" I snap, frustration slipping through the cracks of emotion in my voice. I feel so violated, once again. But then, before I can register what is happening, he reaches down and grabs my foot, like it's the most natural thing in the world. I pull back without thinking, like my body is wired to react that way to touch now. My skin crawls. He's crossed a line; a line I didn't even realize I'd drawn so fiercely until this moment. But that's what happens after you've been through hell—after you've spent months of having your body poked, prodded, tested, and examined by too many hands—even if they are well-meaning. I'm guarded. No one touches me now. No one, except for doctors. And even that is only out of necessity, because I have no other choice. My family knows better. They know the rules, the unspoken ones I've laid out after trauma has made my body into more of a battlefield, than a home.

"I went through some of your medical records," he says casually, straightening up and putting his offending hand back in his pocket. We had given him access to a portion of my medical records, trusting that he was genuinely trying to help us. "Honestly, I was surprised by how little there was. I've worked on big cases and there's just not a lot there."

I stare at him, words of defense stuck in my throat. My eyes dart to my dad's with a silent plea of help.

"Here's my recommendation. Whatever my insurance company offers you, just take it and let's settle this thing out of court. There's no need to go down that road." He looks at me, and then over to mom and dad. I can see the stress and exhaustion spread over both of their faces. They stay silent and direct their stares back at me.

Susan finally steps in, her voice softer than usual, she is almost apologetic in her tone. "I think that's enough for today." She takes Richard's arm in her hand and gives it a gentle tug.

You could cut the tension with a knife. My dad remains in the corner, grinding his teeth, clenching his fists, breathing heavily, trying to remain calm. If I know him, and I do—I know he's a second away from losing it.

"We've taken enough of your time," Richard says, trying to smooth things over. "We just wanted to check in on Caitlin, and we are glad to see she is doing so well."

We exchange strained goodbyes, but Dad doesn't say a word. I know he's holding back biting remarks. And then, just like that, the door closes, and the dust of his words are still swirling.

I can hear the sauce bubbling on the stovetop in the next room.

We sit in silence, trying to process what just went down.

"What was that?" I ask out loud, even though I know we all know the answer. *Why all this charade?* I recall the moment in my hospital room that he pulled my dad aside and urged us to sue. Then, there's the incident where Dave admitted his dad had told him to document my recovery with a video camera, and now this? He just barges in, subjects me to an interrogation, and then dismisses our case based on what he calls a "small" stack of medical records.

I fume as I think about the boxes that have taken up residence in the corner of the living room. They are filled to the brim with medical records from two years ago. The stack is far from small—and they are overflowing with proof. Yet beneath my anger, I feel a pang of sympathy for Richard and Susan. I understand that everything they're doing stems from a desperate attempt to protect their son.

Part of me is relieved. Maybe I don't have a case. Maybe I'm not as broken as everyone thinks I am. Isn't that what I crave? To be normal? To be whole? To be healed? Yet, I know, with every pack of frozen peas I place on my backside, and every pain pill I throw down my throat, that I am far from normal; and healing is a destination to which I still have not been given a map.

I had spent months visualizing myself at my cousin's wedding, twirling on two legs that actually worked, free from pain, laughing and dancing with my family for the first time since the accident. That vision had gotten me through so many long and painful nights. But the reality left me alone, in the corner of the reception, glued to my wheelchair. I had so many plans! I was supposed to hike the Grand Canyon from rim to rim with my best friend for our senior trip. Instead, I am barely able to walk from the bathroom to my bed without feeling like I am going to collapse.

No, I most certainly had a case.

Dad's pacing again, muttering something I can't make out, under his breath.

He leaves the room, phone in hand, already calling someone. Knowing him, he's calling everyone he trusts, trying to make sense of this mess by asking his trusted advisors' opinions.

Mom stays silent, and watches me as I sit there, my young twenty-four-year-old self still trying to wrap my head around what just happened.

"It felt like he didn't believe me," I finally say out loud to the entire room. "The way he grabbed my foot . . ."

Mom exhales a deep, weary sigh. "Cait," she says, looking at me steadily, "most people can't even fathom the hell we've walked through as a family for the last two years, nor can they fully grasp the invisible battles you face every day."

Feeling the need to lighten the mood, I chuckle as I suggest, "Maybe I should attach my X-rays to my back," I joke bitterly. "That would shut them up."

"Not a bad idea," she replies, as we both recall how my pain management doctor looked at those same X-rays a few weeks after my accident and said only, "Holy shit."

I didn't think I'd ever be the type of person to sue anyone. Growing up in a conservative Christian home, I was taught that lawsuits were something to avoid, that grace was the answer, not conflict. Suing someone seems like vengeance or materialism— things that never sat right with my beliefs. We are supposed to solve our problems quietly, without dragging them into the public or making them into something bigger. But this is big. My quality of life is on the line. There's also a guilt that weighs heavily on me. I've met so many wonderful people in therapy and during my hospital stays. It feels selfish sometimes to think I deserve compensation when others are suffering just as much, if not more. But I never imagined my life would change this drastically. I never thought pain would become the center of everything, that my body would betray me like this, draining me of energy, of life. But here I am, on the verge of it, and I still can't quite believe it. The whole idea feels foreign, like it belongs to someone else's life, not mine. I am not the kind of person who throws lawyers at people, who demands compensation for my own pain. But then again, I never thought I'd be the kind of person who couldn't walk through a store for ten minutes without having to locate the nearest bench. When your life falls apart in the way mine has, things are no longer black and white. They get gray very, very fast.

*　　*　　*

It's been over two years since the accident—over two years of relentless, debilitating pain, isolation, immobility, and pretending I'm fine when I'm anything but. My dad and I weave through traffic, trying to make it to the appointment on time, but I'm lost in thought as I stare out the window. I'm still stuck in yesterday, when my brother had to carry me out of Hobby Lobby. My legs just quit on me halfway through the store, and I looked at him, panicked, searching for anywhere to sit.

"Cait, look at you," he had snapped, frustration and concern sharpening his voice as he lifted me from the Hobby Lobby floor like I was his baby sister again. "You need to do this. You deserve to be compensated for all this pain."

My brother's words echo in my head as my dad and I enter the lawyer's office—this big, imposing building at the center of town, all glass and steel. It feels too formal, which means it must all be too real. My brother is right, though, even if I don't want to admit it. I can barely sit upright without waves of pain coursing through me; it feels like I am being stabbed in my tailbone over and over again.

I take a seat, sinking into my black donut cushion, my constant companion as I examine the men in black suits seated along the long, polished conference table. Their faces are serious as they discuss my case like it is just another Tuesday. For them, maybe it is. Another day, another broken person walking into their office, trying to piece their life back together. I suspect they're all lawyers, or at least part of the legal team, though it's difficult to say for certain.

I know one thing—I don't want to be here, in this room with the mix of leather and cologne hanging in the air. I can feel the memories of Dave and the accident pressing at the edges of my mind, fraying my forgetfulness. I had fought so hard to bury them, but now they are rising to the surface of my memory like ghosts that refuse to stay dead.

I feel my body begin to shake with the force of the emotion and as I try slowing down my breathing, I beg God to help me conceal how nervous I am. The door swings open and an older gentleman enters the room; his presence is commanding yet unassuming. He takes his place at the head of the table. My chair, edged right next to him, feels both too close and yet exactly where I need to be, even if I don't want it. His eyes catch mine, and I can tell right away they are a seasoned lawyer's eyes, but they are not the cold, calculating ones I had braced myself for. Instead, his warm smile disarms me, and I can feel myself start to sag with involuntary relief.

He reaches out, hand extended. "Pleased to meet you," he says, his voice smooth and surprisingly gentle, so far from the formidable figure I had imagined.

I look down at the small cooler resting beside me, crammed with ice packs. My survival kit. The only thing standing between me and another handful of pain pills. I catch a few glances flicker toward it, like they're trying to figure out what I'm carrying around with me. Maybe they'll just assume it's my lunch.

The voices around me start to blur, becoming distant echoes as I zone out. I answer their questions on autopilot, not really present, not really there. It's like everything is moving in slow motion, like I am watching it all happen from somewhere outside my own body. Hours pass—hours filled with rehashing the accident, the pain, the aftermath. I feel drained, completely empty.

"Caitlin, are you listening?" My dad's voice pulls me back.

I blink and nod, forcing myself to focus. "Yes," I say, though it doesn't feel like I am really there, not fully.

My dad's old friend sits to my left, a small comfort in this sea of unfamiliar faces. He's been helping us through this mess, guiding us, trying to figure out how to move forward. His presence has been reassuring.

Then, one of the lawyers speaks, and the mood shifts.

"Did you know Dave's father ordered the car from the accident to be destroyed just three days after it happened?"

"Destroyed?" My dad responds before I can even process this new information. "No, we didn't know that," he states steadily.

The lawyer continues, laying it out like it was nothing. "He made sure there was no evidence left behind."

I am stunned, trying to wrap my head around what I am hearing. But it's not over. He has more information to share.

"We also found out Dave was drug tested at the first hospital you were taken to, but there's no trace of those results. Just gone, like they never existed. It's pretty clear something happened to them. What exactly? We may never know."

I don't say anything—just shake my head in disbelief, staring at my cooler of frozen peas.

"We did some deeper digging on Dave," the lawyer went on, his voice calm. "One of the top private investigators in the country uncovered a long history of reckless driving and abuse. Apparently, he beat up one girl so badly, he was banned from his college campus. And you're not the first person he's injured in a car accident. There's another girl walking around with injuries similar to yours."

My stomach churns. I feel like I can't breathe. "I'm sorry, what?!" I manage to say, my voice shaking.

But the lawyer just keeps going, like this is just another piece of the puzzle that he wants me to finish right then and there. Another fact to add to the pile. Shock overtakes me and my dad has to take over the duty of listening. I zone out and trust that he is taking in every word. He's been my biggest advocate through all of this, fighting for me when I didn't have the strength to fight for myself; documenting everything, making calls, doing whatever he could to make sure I was taken care of.

"You've been lied to, Caitlin," the lawyer says, his voice gentler now, almost pitying. "He played you. He told you to settle with his insurance, take whatever they offered, because he knows damn well you're entitled to a whole lot more. And he's counting on you not figuring that out."

I leave the building, my mind going a thousand different directions. Abused women. Car accidents. Destroyed evidence.

How had I missed this? How had I been so blind? The guilt hits me hard—guilt for staying with him, for letting him have so much control over my life. For believing, even for a second, that things could have been different.

My dad steadies me as I sink into the car, every part of me weighed down by a bone-deep weariness that is etched across my face.

"We are doing this and seeing it through," Dad says with a confidence I am simply too tired to grasp. I nod, too exhausted to say a word.

I half-listen as he rehashes the plans about my lawyers in Florida partnering with a nationally-renowned lawyer from Texas, a man who only takes on a few cases each year. "The odds are slim," he admits. I nod, barely able to speak. "Okay," I whisper.

We pull into my parents' driveway; the engine idles and neither one of us moves to get out of the car. My chest tightens. Stress—in whatever shape it takes—always magnifies the pain. The only thing I can think about now is crawling into bed, burying myself beneath the ice packs and shutting out the world.

The door cracks open, and there is Mom, standing on the porch, already in full interrogation mode. The questions start immediately: What happened at the meeting? What did they say? How was I feeling? I stare back for a few seconds, trying to make my mind form a sentence but realize I don't remember much of what was said at the meeting. Not really. Other than a few sharp points about Dave—his dad destroying the car, the things they'd dug up about his past—I can't recall a single detail. It's like my brain shut off the moment I stepped into that sterile conference room. Maybe it was some sort of defense mechanism; self-preservation kicking in, shutting down to avoid the pain of reliving it all. Or maybe it was the pain pills. Or both.

"I can't do this right now," I finally manage to say. "I just want this all to go away. I don't even want to pursue the lawsuit. I don't think I can handle the stress."

Mom doesn't miss a beat. She is compassionate and firm. "Cait, we don't know what your future looks like. It's been over two years since your accident, and you can barely get out of bed most days. And when you do, you're so drugged up you can hardly function."

Like I need the reminder. Like I wasn't already painfully aware that my body, my life, had become a prison. Her words stung in that way only a mother's can, not because they were untrue, but because they were too true. They were the things I tried not to think about, the truths I buried under layers of denial just so I could try to make it through the day.

"I can't talk anymore," I snap at her, more harshly than I mean to, and storm down the hall to my room.

I sit down on the edge of my bed and try to peel off my shirt, desperate to slip into something more comfortable. But even reaching for the soft cotton T-shirt I have been living in feels like a challenge. The constriction of my bra is unbearable; it feels like someone has wrapped me in barbed wire, and I can't get it off fast enough. I try to pull the fabric over my head, but my arms won't cooperate; the muscles are too weak and I am too sore. I had resorted to having Botox injected into my back, neck, and shoulders because paralyzing the muscles was supposed to stop the spasms that would leave me so debilitated I could do nothing but lie down.

Struggling to extricate myself from my shirt, I feel the familiar tiny tingle, it's like my nerves are warning me. They know before I do that the spasms are coming. And with them, a wave of anxiety that's almost worse than the pain itself washes over me. Botox sounded like a good idea at the time, but now? Now, I can barely move my arms. My pain management doctor says I am covered in scar tissue—it's everywhere, tangled in the muscles that had been ripped apart in the accident, like jagged shards of glass. The way he'd said it, it was so matter-of-fact. I've tried every injection known to man, and still, nothing provides real relief.

My face has swollen so much from the steroids they pumped into me that I barely recognize myself when I look in the mirror. I googled it once—apparently, it's called "moon face." Fitting, in the most awful way. I had hit my max dose of steroids for the year. And the pain never really goes away, driving me to the edge some days. So much so that I'd take the smooth side of a butter knife and press it into my muscles, violently digging in, desperate to release the tension, the pressure, the painful knots. I keep going until bruises bloom, deep purple and blue patches, ugly reminders of my desperation to find relief. My friend, whose eyes were wide with horror after she took in the bruises scattered across my body, purchased me a blue rolling device, made for people with chronic pain. Same idea as the butter knife, just a gentler approach. It helps some but offers only temporary relief at best.

I pull the gel ice packs and frozen peas from the cooler, one by one, and arrange them across the bed, mapping out the worst of the pain. Then, before lying down, I grab the butter knife and press it into the knots that have twisted up inside me from the day. The mirror catches my leg's reflection—broken capillaries, bruises popping up beneath the surface. It's painful but I grit my teeth and keep rubbing. One after another. I don't care. I just need it to stop.

I never could have guessed that one day, the same butter knife and that cheap blue roller device would be laid out in front of a room full of sharply dressed strangers, revealing only a small snapshot into my private struggle.

FIFTEEN

SUICIDE DISEASE

Trying to explain chronic pain feels like describing a color no one else can see. It wears me down and pulls at my sanity until I question if I'm still tethered to reality. I'm moving more now—walking unassisted for minutes at a time—and people seem to think that means everything's better. I thought it would too. I thought walking meant I'd feel normal again, like I'd finally won. But every day is still a battle in the war I am waging with my own body. Chronic pain is cruel like that—it tears you apart from the inside, leaving no visible scars, nothing for the world to see, but you feel it all.

*   *   *

The turquoise journal wasn't anything special when I first bought it—just an ordinary notebook, its pages blank and waiting, with a calendar I never thought I'd need. I didn't expect it to become something important, that it would sit witness to some of the most important parts of my story. Now, more than two years later, it's filled with victories I never imagined I'd have to track, the kind of milestones no one prepares you for. I call them microgoals.

Stood for five minutes today holding onto my walker.

Worked out arms with dumbbells in the wheelchair.

Graduated pool therapy.

I drove my mom's car today around the neighborhood, with my dad in the passenger seat, while using my left leg. Next up—overcome fear of driving on the main roads.

May 7, 2012: I can now do the elliptical with the assistance of a band around my waist, while my therapist holds the back of the band keeping me steady. I worked up to ten minutes today. I could only do about thirty seconds when I first started a month ago. I was forced to stop when the nerve pain became too intense. They had to ice the entire lower half of my body afterward. I'd be lying if I said the pain is not getting to me.

When you live in pain—the debilitating kind of chronic pain—day after day, time becomes blurry. It's like living in a fog where everything bleeds together, and you forget where one day ends and the next begins. You start to lose track of progress. Am I getting anywhere? Or am I just a body, locked in place while the world moves on without me?

That's why I write it all down. Without these notes, these records of the small steps forward, I'm afraid I'll lose sight of any movement at all. Some days, it feels like I'm moving in slow motion, dragging this broken body of mine through each moment. Other days, I'm just standing still, waiting for something to change.

But then I flip through these pages and see it—the proof. I am still moving.

Today, I tried cooking again. Not just throwing together a turkey and pickle sandwich with a dab of mayo and mustard, but an actual meal—something that requires real effort. Cooking was always my thing, a kind of art I inherited from my dad, who has been our family's personal chef for as long as I can remember. After the accident, though, I let that part of me go. I let others step in, take over cooking, bringing me meals because I couldn't manage on my own.

It's noon. I decide to make a pizza for lunch—a modest, homemade attempt at normalcy. But ten minutes in, the nerves along my spine start flaring up, angry and relentless. I feel my muscles twist into painful knots, and I know my time is running short. I am not about to give up though. I grab an Ace bandage off the countertop, having placed it there because I knew at some point I would need it. I wrap it tightly around my back to secure the large gel ice pack in place. Once the dough is rolled, I feel the deep burn of my sciatic nerve shooting down my right leg into my big toe. I quickly shift my weight to my left leg, the leg I now favor, as I sort of balance myself against the countertop with my left elbow. I awkwardly dice up veggies and add the cheese and pepperonis to the pizza dough, the ice numbing me just enough to muscle through these last steps. *Finally*. Pizza is in the oven. I set the timer and head for my room to lie down.

The timer beeps, and the smell of pizza drifts into my bedroom. I push myself up, making my way to the kitchen where I pull the pizza from the oven. I swap out my ice pack—the old one already warm and useless—and sit at the table on my black donut cushion. It's stained and fraying at the edges, worn down from too many days spent planted in the same spot. I eat almost the entire pizza by myself, my mind drifting, before heading back to bed, to the fortress of pillows that's become my world. I grab my TENS unit, a portable muscle stimulator that helps with pain relief, lay out my ice packs, and collapse.

The layers of ice packs press against my skin as I drift into sleep. When I wake, it's not the usual ache that prompts my eyes open, but a sharp, deep pain in my back that jolts me upright. I head to the full-length mirror and there it is: An ice burn, dark and angry, seared into the right side of my back. Permanent, maybe. I panic, grab my phone, and google the remedy. A warm compress, it says. I shuffle into the kitchen, grab a dishcloth, and run it under warm water, the sting of the burn pulsing in my back. As I press it to my skin, I hear her voice behind me.

"What are you doing, Cait?" my mom asks.

"Nothing, Mom, don't worry about it," I say quickly, trying to sidestep the inevitable lecture. I make my way back to my room, avoiding her eyes, knowing full well she'd tell me not to put the ice directly on my skin.

Somehow mom talks me into attending a family gathering at my aunt and uncle's house this evening, even though I don't feel like going anywhere. I leave the ice packs, Ace bandages, and TENS unit behind, determined to pretend, just for a little while, that I don't need them.

I sit on the couch most of the evening, trying to keep up with the conversation, nodding at all the right moments, but my mind is elsewhere. All I can think about is how I should've brought my ice packs. We stay longer than I expected—hours, actually—and the pain intensifies. I excuse myself again, heading to the bathroom where I pop more oxycodone than I care to admit. I keep the little orange bottle hidden at the bottom of my purse, in a small makeup pouch. I try to conceal it as best as I can, so that no one knows. I'm not proud of it, but I just need to feel human long enough to get through this, to make it through one more conversation without wincing. I look at myself in the mirror, swallow hard, and wonder how much longer I can keep pretending. I just want to be normal. To have something real to say when people ask me what I'm doing with my life. But instead, I offer them a smile, the kind that's practiced, the kind that stops the conversation from going too deep. I don't want anyone to know about the pain and my overall health and just how debilitated I am.

And then there's the lawsuit—a constant shadow, making me feel like I'm being watched, waiting for someone to call me a liar, to accuse me again that the pain isn't real. I've turned into a ghost, haunting the corners of my own home, staying isolated from the outside world—I need to feel protected. But I can't stop thinking about how foolish I was to believe I'd be better by now, that somehow, life would snap back to what it used to be. Normal? Normal is a fantasy, a cruel trick of memory. Yes, I've made progress. But at a pace so slow it feels like I'm moving backward, like I'll never catch up. And I can't accept this as my life. I won't.

Grief still comes in waves, and today I feel like I'm drowning in it. The undertow of denial keeps pulling me under, still searching for answers that don't exist, still chasing medications that offer nothing but empty promises and more disappointment.

I've been researching spinal cord stimulators as an alternative to pain medications, and now I find myself in a top pain management clinic, clutching at the possibility of something—anything—that can break the cycle.

I sit on the crinkled paper of the exam table, shifting my weight every few minutes. When Dr. Green walks in, I can tell right away this is not going to be a productive appointment. He doesn't even make eye contact.

"What brings you in today?" he asks, glancing at the stack of folders on his desk. He looks bored.

I try to hold back the frustration I'm feeling, but before I know it the words just spill out.

"I'm in chronic pain every day, all day, and I need help," I manage to say, my voice trembling.

"Where does it hurt?"

He hasn't even looked at my chart.

"My whole body," I answer, trying to keep my voice steady.

"Well," he says, barely glancing up, "We don't just hand out painkillers these days. Have you tried ibuprofen? Maybe alternate with Tylenol?"

That's it. The switch flips. He thinks I'm just here for the drugs. I can feel the anger rising up in me.

"I'm not here for pain medications!" The words explode out of me, louder than I intend them to.

Dr. Green looks up, startled. His eyes widen.

"I was ejected from a car over two years ago. Spent six months in a hospital bed, and you'd know that if you'd even glanced at my medical records. I look fine, yeah, but I'm not. I hate taking those damn pain pills, but I need something—anything—to make it through. I'm not here for more drugs. I'm here for an alternative. Can you help me or not?" I hold his gaze and with my stare I communicate what I can't manage to say out loud: I've been through the wringer and you are my last hope.

He pauses, then does something I don't expect. He smiles. I feel taken aback and look down at my bum leg. "Well, you're not your average bear, are you?" he says, settling onto his stool. "This is the most refreshing appointment I've had in a while."

I blink. Look back at him, stunned.

We sit in silence for a few moments before I speak again, my voice softer now.

"I want to know more about spinal stimulators. I read something about them helping with chronic pain online. I'm also open to other recommendations you may have."

He nods. "Sure. I can set you up with a consult to go over it, but I'll be honest—it's usually something we use for elderly patients. And the success rate isn't high."

I feel deflated. Of course, it's never that simple.

"What else is there?" I ask, my voice desperate as I try to keep the tears at bay. "I'm forced to take oxycodone anytime I want to do something as simple as just dinner with a friend. The pain is so debilitating." My voice trails off, conveying the hopelessness I feel.

Dr. Green leans in a bit. "Well, there's a new medication—a time-released morphine. It might help for longer outings or, possibly, weaning off the oxycodone altogether."

I hesitate, but only for a second. Anything to get off the oxy. "Okay, I'll try it," I blurt out in frustration. I know I have no other option.

He flips through my medical charts and then walks over to examine my leg. "Can I check your leg and foot? The one with nerve damage?"

I shift again, my body aching. "Sure."

He gently lifts my leg, treating it like delicate glass, inspecting it with careful attention. "Can you move your ankle at all?"

"I can now wiggle my toes."

He nods. "That's good. Means the nerves are still firing." He pauses. "Is it always this blue and purple?"

"Most of the time, especially after I've been walking."

"Has anyone mentioned CRPS to you?" he asks, eyes narrowing as he studies my leg some more.

"No," I answer. "What's that?"

"Complex regional pain syndrome," he says, like it's a common phrase, something you'd hear at the grocery store or on a subway. "In your case, it was caused by trauma to the nerves from the accident. These small nerve fibers are transmitting severe pain signals. It can cause temperature changes and discoloration in the affected area. Some people can barely stand a light touch on their skin. From everything I'm seeing, you're a textbook case."

CRPS. It's a name, *finally*. A label for the monster I've been fighting for so long. It's like I've been handed an answer, something to point at and say, "This is it. This is what's been wrecking me."

"Not many doctors are familiar with it. This is the third case I've seen this year." Dr. Green sighs as he looks at me carefully. "I'll be the first to tell you—it's not in your head. You're not crazy. And this condition is incredibly difficult to manage, let alone treat."

I nod intently, feeling the tears press behind my eyes, burning, but I force them to stay where they are, as I think of the nights when a bedsheet brushing against my foot was enough to make me want to scream. *I'm not crazy—the pain isn't just in my head.*

I feel like a weight has been lifted, only to be replaced by a new one—heavier, crushing, just in a different way. But at least now I know. At least now I have a doctor's assurance that I'm not losing my mind. Dr. Green slides a few papers toward me.

"Here's everything you'll need. Talk to your family, make sure they know what's going on. You're going to need a strong support system."

"I've got one, and I wouldn't still be here without them."

He gives me a small smile, standing up. "Hang in there. We'll set up another appointment soon, see how you're responding to the new meds."

I nod and start perusing the papers. "Thanks."

Then, just before he leaves, I ask the question that's been clawing at me. I can't leave without getting an answer. "Is there a cure?"

Dr. Green pauses, lowers his head for a moment, and then looks back at me. "No. I'm sorry."

Somehow, I already knew that. A gut feeling maybe.

For the next week or so, I spend most of my waking hours researching CRPS. I treat learning about this condition like it's my job. I want to know everything I can about it so I can conquer it.

I learn it is most commonly referred to as the "suicide disease" because, well, that makes a lot of sense.

I watch videos on YouTube of people sharing about their experience with CRPS. Our stories are so similar yet different in some ways. My condition was triggered by a direct injury to the nerve, while tragically, for others, the cause may be unknown. I quickly realize that it's a rare disease and there's still not a lot known about how to go about treating it.

My friends are coming over tonight to watch a movie, which is exactly what I need. Something to take my mind off all the research and dead ends. We try to do this every weekend and it's a time I have come to look forward to all week. I cherish the company and conversation. I decide to try out the time-released morphine for the first time; I'm a bit nervous because I've reacted poorly to a number of medications given to me in the past for nerve pain. I chug down the pill with a glass of water and lean back into the recliner.

My friends arrive, and soon we're laughing, trading stories, passing around chips and dip, and then heading into the kitchen for the ice cream. I find myself surprised as the movie plays on—no need to reach for an ice pack or heating pad, no rotating from side to side every couple of minutes, no sharp reminder of pain interrupting the moment. For the first time in a while, I let myself hope—maybe this is going to work out after all.

I start taking the morphine daily, and at first, it's like someone finally turned the volume down on my pain. I feel relief—real relief. I marvel at the lack of pain when I wake up in the morning. I forgot what that felt like. It's enough to bring me to tears. But by week two, the morphine stops working, or maybe my body just stops responding. The pain creeps back in, and I'm so tired. More tired than I thought was possible. I barely have the strength to drag myself out of bed, and I don't even try most days. I just sit here, staring at the wall, feeling the hours tick by without caring. I don't want to talk. I don't want to move. I can't remember the last time I showered. I feel like a zombie moving through the motions without any spark of life left inside me.

I can't do this anymore, I decide. I can't keep riding this endless cycle of meds, chasing temporary moments of relief. The pain always comes back. And when it does, it hits harder, digs deeper, like it's learned something new about how to hurt me. I can feel my body giving up—like something inside me is slowly decaying, each pill pulls me further away from who I used to be. The years of chronic stress, pain, and drugs are eating me alive. My muscles, once strong, are now soft and I feel useless.

It's like I've been poisoned, and I'm always going to feel sick and hollowed out. My body is shutting down, piece by piece, part by part, and I don't know how to stop it.

SIXTEEN

ROCK BOTTOM

It's the dead of the night when I jolt awake, my heart pounding so hard it feels like it's trying to break through my ribs. *What is happening?* I try to turn over, pressing my hands against the pillows to push myself up, but my body won't respond. My limbs are heavy and useless as I fall back into the mattress. Panic shoots through me as I try to yell out for my mom, but the words come out thick and slurred, getting caught on my swollen tongue. *Am I dying? Is this what a heart attack feels like?* I wonder as my fear overwhelms me.

I can't lie here waiting for answers, because I'm sure if I do, I'm going to die. The bed feels miles from the floor, but somehow, I manage to roll myself to the edge, throwing pillows onto the floor in some half-hearted attempt to soften the fall. I tumble down with a thud, my knees buckling the moment they hit the mountain of pillows. I'm too disoriented to even notice the pain. The room spins violently around me, every movement sending waves of nausea through my body, but I force myself to crawl. My hands scrape against the thick fibers of the carpet, as I inch my way toward my parents' room.

I reach the side of my dad's bed first, grab onto the comforter, and yank with what little strength I have left. "Dad," I croak, the sound barely escaping my lips.

He bolts upright, fumbling for the light switch, panic flooding his eyes as he looks at me crumpled on the floor. Mom is awake now too, hovering behind him.

"What's wrong?" he asks as he crouches down next to me.

"I think . . . I'm having a heart attack," I slur.

In one swift motion, he scoops me up and carries me like I'm a child, out into the night, and gently eases me onto the passenger seat of his truck, my body slumping against the door. Mom climbs into the backseat, and I feel her hand, warm and comforting, on my shoulder. She doesn't say anything, but I know she's trying to hold it together. Dad drives like a bat out of hell, breaking every speed limit, the tires squealing with each turn, as we make our way to the emergency room.

At the ER, they don't waste any time. The only words that needed to be spoken come from my dad: "She thinks she's having a heart attack." That's all it took. In seconds, they have me in a hospital bed. I barely have time to blink before I am covered in wires.

The ER doctor on call bolts through the door. "What happened?"

"We don't know!" Dad rattles off my meds list, the history spilling out in fragments.

A nurse pierces my skin with needles, drawing blood after blood; it's as if they are attempting to siphon answers from my veins. I drift in and out of consciousness, the relentless beeping of the heart monitor screeching every few minutes. My pulse plummets, then spikes out of nowhere, the machine blares a warning as nurses rush in repeatedly.

I have no idea how long I've been lying here—time's a blur. It could be an hour, maybe more. Finally, the doctor steps back in.

"Her bloodwork's back. Caitlin has dangerously high serotonin levels. It's serotonin syndrome."

"What does that even mean?" Mom asks the doctor without taking her eyes off of me.

The doctor nods at me and asks, "Have you started any new medications? You mentioned oxycodone and a few others for pain."

I struggle to find my voice. My tongue is less swollen now, but I'm still so sluggish. "Yeah . . . I am on a time-released morphine pill."

The doctor sighs, and it's the kind of sound that tells you everything you don't want to know. "That's it. The dose mixed with your other meds is what most likely caused this. You need to stop taking it immediately. We don't want you to go into congestive heart failure. Patients typically have to be intubated with serotonin syndrome. You are lucky," he says as he looks down at me sympathetically.

It all makes sense now, like the pieces of a dangerous, messed-up puzzle falling into place. Before I have time to fully process everything, the nurse is hooking me up to an IV. I feel the cold fluid rushing through my veins, flushing out the toxins. I focus on keeping still, but the pain is all-consuming. I can't take anything else for it—my body's reached its limit. Mom can see right through me, the way I'm struggling to hold on. She leans in and whispers to the nurse, asking if they can make me some ice packs.

Minutes later, I feel her gentle hands sliding the ice beneath my neck, along my spine, and under my tailbone. *Relief.*

I spend the night fading in and out of sleep.

By morning, they check my vitals and then send me home, like I am just another number to check off their list. Walking into my parents' house, I am hit with a wave of emotions. *I'm not living. I am simply surviving. Barely.*

"Dad," I whisper, "If I don't make a change, I'm going to die. I can't do this anymore."

My parents just stand there, their silence saying everything words can't. Because what was there to say? There aren't words for this kind of brokenness. I can feel their helplessness echoing my own. None of us know which way to turn anymore, where to find help. Dad hugs me, doing his best to reassure me that everything will be okay.

I turn slowly, each step heavy as I walk back to my room and close the door behind me, defeated.

I sleep through most of the day, drifting in and out of this surreal fog that clings, unwilling to lift. Everything's blurred at the edges, as if I'm looking through a thick pane of glass.

Did I really drag myself to my parents' room last night, convinced I was dying?

The memories are slippery now and I can't hold onto them—faint flashes of the hospital, the nurses in their baby-blue scrubs, the machines that kept beeping endlessly. It's all so jumbled together. And somehow, it already feels distant, like it happened to someone else entirely.

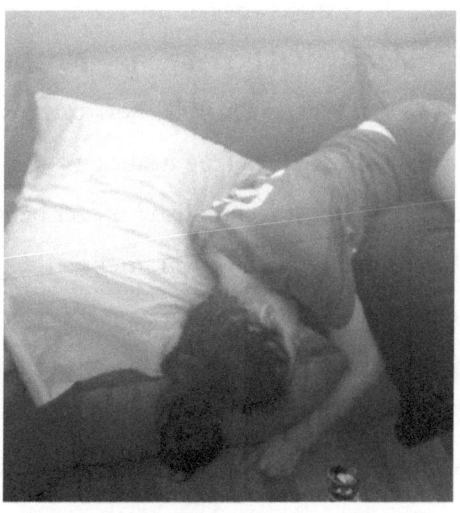

My emotions have been a mess throughout this whole thing, spiraling in ways I didn't even think were possible. I've been depressed before—more times than I'd like to admit. But this . . . this is different. It's like a black hole, swallowing me up, pulling me under so deep that there's no light to see, there is no hope to hold onto so that I can catch my breath at the surface.

The depression is not gentle, not something that creeps into my awareness subtly— it's a full-body collapse, drowning me from the inside out, making it hard to breathe, to think, to care about anything in what is left of my life. I feel it in my bones, in the pit of my stomach, crushing me until there's nothing left. I want nothing more than to curl up in the safety of my bed, to become a tightly wound ball of nothingness and hide from the world.

* * *

Night has quietly settled in. I glance over at the pill bottles lined up on the black shelf in the corner of my room, their labels facing forward at attention, like soldiers awaiting orders. I've stared at them too many times. New pain pills, new promises. But now I know better—they can't fix me. True healing is not going to come in the form of a pill. I almost feel foolish for ever believing it could.

For a brief, gut-wrenching moment, the thought cuts through my heart like a knife: *I could end it all right now.* Just one choice and it'd be over. You hear about it, see it in movies—people swallowing a bottle of pills and slipping away.

I slide out of bed, every inch of my body aching. I grab the nearest bottle—an orange one, deceptively small and deadly in its promise of relief. I grip the bottle, my fingers digging into its smooth plastic surface, staring hard at it. It's like holding a grenade, heavy with the weight of what's inside, and what it could do. I flip the cap on and off, the soft click filling the quiet room. Each time the cap comes off, I imagine what it would be like to swallow them all, to finally let go, to let everything just . . . fade away, to be finished with the crippling pain, fatigue, and depression. I want to shut it all out . . . to feel nothing.

But something from deep inside stops me, keeping my hand from tipping those tiny pills past my lips, taking me into oblivion. It's not a grand revelation, not some earth-shattering moment of clarity. It's small, so small, it's barely there. But I catch it; a glimmer of hope, because if I'm honest, there's a part of me that still wants to live, that still believes maybe, just maybe, I could get my life back. It's faint, fragile even, but it's enough to keep my hand from twisting the cap open one last time. It's enough to keep me alive.

Angrily, I throw the bottle against the wall, watching as it breaks open, scattering pills across the floor like the broken pieces of my life. Then, the sobs come. Deep, and guttural, they tear through me as tears blur my vision and I collapse into my bed, my body shaking.

"God, please help me," I whisper into the emptiness. I say it again, and again, until my voice is ragged, and my body is hollowed out from the weight of it all.

I use a pillow to wipe the tears from my face and notice my Bible lying on my nightstand, resting under my lamp, as if it's been waiting for me. I don't even know what I'm searching for, but I open it anyway, my fingers instinctively turning to the Psalms. Psalm 61 stares back at me: "When my heart is overwhelmed, lead me to the rock that is higher than I."

I read it out loud, the words both foreign and familiar on my tongue. And then I keep reading, my voice trembling as I go. I read some of the verses twice, maybe more, as if the repetition might pull me back from the edge.

In this moment of rawness, I feel it all—the shattered pieces of everything with Dave, the crushing guilt and shame of the accident that almost took my life. I think about the last two years, how they've slipped through my fingers, wasted on pain and loss. It feels like a black hole of time, swallowed up by suffering. But maybe, just maybe, it wasn't all for nothing. Maybe there's meaning buried somewhere in this mess of hurt. Maybe I lived for a reason.

I close the Bible and just hold it, pressing it tightly against my chest. Minutes go by. Then, something shifts inside me. It's not sudden, not the kind of lightning-bolt moment I thought it would be. It's slow, like warmth creeping into my frozen bones, filling the spaces that have been empty for so long. For the first time in what seems like forever, I'm feeling something other than pain. It's Jesus. Soft, steady, like an embrace—wrapping itself around me. It's like being hugged by someone who sees every piece of me, all the broken fragments and doesn't look away. It feels like a father's hug, the way he would comfort a child who's been lost and is hurting. I feel a peace that doesn't make sense to me, in the middle of all this chaos. And it's certainly not the kind that wipes everything clean or makes the hurt disappear. But for the first time, I look at the accident, the pain, Dave—all of it—and I see it differently. Like every bit of it has been working together for my good, pulling me out of the toxic wreckage of that relationship. Maybe even rescuing me from myself. I've been beaten down, broken down, physically, mentally, emotionally. But for the first time in a long while, my heart softens.

Tears flow, and with them, the bitterness, the emptiness, and the shame start to drain away.

I cry for everything that has been lost, but within that sorrow there's a budding sense of gratitude for even the pain itself. The rough edges of it have carved into me, molded me into something new, something harder and softer all at once. I cling to the scripture reference my mom recited to me in the trauma ICU, her voice steady but her eyes barely recognizing the battered body of her child: "All things work together for good." Again, in the rehab hospital, she repeated it like a prayer, like some lifeline that was going to rescue me out of that situation. I didn't want to hear it then. I wanted to scream at her to stop. But now, I get it. This verse offers a message of hope and assurance that, despite the challenges and pains of life, there is a divine purpose at work.

It suggests that there is good in even the most difficult circumstances. I don't necessarily view my suffering as good, but rather it could be used in a transformative way—for my own growth, to build a deeper faith, and perhaps even be used to help others through similar trials. It allows me to trust in a bigger plan and know that I am being shaped and guided for purposes that align with divine love and wisdom.

* * *

It's been two days since I got home from the hospital, but the scare of serotonin syndrome still lingers in my thoughts. I feel sick, like I'm battling the flu and a hangover all at once. My body aches, pain slashing through every inch of me. But somewhere beneath all the pain is a trace of hope. Hope, even after everything. It's quiet, almost imperceptible, but it's there. I have this feeling that I can get through this. But I'm not naïve, I know what's coming—it's going to get worse before it even thinks about getting better. I've danced through the horrors of medication withdrawal before and it's never a graceful exit.

Mom sits on the sectional, while I'm on the opposite end, my legs stretched out and propped up on a pile of pillows.

"This is it. I'm getting off all of it," I say through tears. "I can't live like this anymore. The medications are slowly killing me."

My mom, hands rubbing her temples, pleads with me, "You need to call your pain management doctor. Please, let's get help this time. The fentanyl withdrawals were so bad. I don't want to watch you go through that again. And you've got so many meds to come off."

I nod, like I get it, but I don't want to hear it. "I'm calling now," I say, grabbing my phone, desperate to take control of something, anything.

I dial the number, hold my breath as it rings. The nurse picks up—finally—and I put it on speaker so my parents can hear.

"Hi, this is Angela, I'm Dr. Green's nurse. How can I help you?"

I fumble over my words, trying to make her understand the desperation in my voice. "I'm on a lot of medications for pain, and they're not working. I feel like I'm dying. I need to get off them—all of them."

She pauses, clicking through my chart, pulling up the mess that's become my medical history. "Well, you definitely don't want to go cold turkey on these. You'll need to taper, slowly, one at a time."

I feel my stomach tighten. *I know this already. I've heard it a hundred times before.* "Is there a rehab facility? Something that can help me through it?"

Another pause, a sigh. "A rehab facility won't take you. You're not an addict."

I almost laugh. *Define addict.* My body sure as hell doesn't care how I got here—it's addicted, whether I chose this or not. But I stay quiet, biting back the urge to scream.

"There are medications to help with withdrawal," she continues, "but you'll need to come in for an evaluation to see if you're a good candidate."

Good candidate?

"Okay," I say, but I already know I'm not making that appointment.

I hang up and toss the phone onto the couch, frustration boiling over.

"Well, that wasn't helpful," I mutter. "She didn't tell me anything I didn't already know." Mom suggests trying another doctor, but I'm done. I'm done with all of it. "No, I'm starting this today, with or without help. I'm doing it. I'm done."

Day one.

I start with Cymbalta—the two-in-one drug, supposed to fix both nerve pain and depression, but it's done neither.

By nightfall, my head is pounding with the worst migraine I've ever experienced. I've had my share of migraines from the accident, but this . . . this is something else. It's like my brain is about to explode from the pressure. I contemplate asking my parents to take me to the ER. Every time I move, I feel these electric zaps that shoot through my skull, and I'm forced to keep my eyes shut.

I slowly reach for my laptop trying not to move my head too much and look it up: Cymbalta withdrawal. Brain zaps. Normal. It could last for weeks.

And it does.

Next, I cut out Lyrica and tramadol.

Then oxycodone and Lortabs.

I also eliminate prescription and over the counter anti-inflammatories that I take daily around the clock.

The withdrawals hit hard. For weeks, I'm curled up in bed, drenched in sweat, vomiting between waves of migraines that feel like they're splitting my skull in two. My mom and sister beg me to slow down, to let my body catch a break. My dad doesn't say much—he knows when my mind's made up, there's no stopping me. I'm stubborn like him in that way.

Three months. Three slow, agonizing months. I try to tell myself it's progress, that I'm making it, inching forward, but it doesn't feel that way. I'm tapering off the meds, or at least trying to. There are moments when I break, when I reach for a tiny dose of those white, circular shaped pills— just enough to take the edge off and make the pain bearable, just enough to feel like I'm not completely losing my mind. Every time I give in and take a pill, it feels like I've failed all over again. Like I'm back at the start.

The withdrawal . . . it's difficult to describe. It's like being trapped in a body that's turned on you. There's this horrible restlessness that takes over. It's like this energy that you can't control—your muscles are twitching under your skin, your bones vibrating. I can't stop moving, can't stop shaking. It's as if my body and mind have disconnected, both going haywire in their own separate ways.

My parents just watch. Helpless. Their eyes say it all—they don't know what to do with me. I don't know what to do with myself either. I'm like some experiment gone wrong, some malfunctioning machine they can't fix. They're waiting for this to end, waiting for me to get better. The only thing that brings any relief to my body is the sun. I sit outside on the wicker lounge chair and let its warmth wash over me. The sun not only soothes me during moments of intense anxiety but also helps ease the burning pain throughout my body.

I get lost in thought when I'm out here gazing up at the bright light in the sky. Sometimes, I let the tears fall, quietly concealed behind a large pair of black sunglasses. Today I think about that doctor in my hometown I saw a few months ago. I sat in his office pleading with him for help—an alternative to painkillers. His solution was to "Pop a pain pill and have a margarita." He chuckled even though he was dead serious, like that would solve all my problems. He treated me like I should be grateful just to be alive. Like surviving this wasn't the hardest thing I'd ever done. I almost wish he had slapped me instead. It would've hurt less.

The pain never stops. It's deep, raw, like every nerve in my body is inflamed. That's the cruel irony of coming off painkillers—the pain doesn't go away, it only intensifies. Lying comfortably is impossible, no matter whether it's day or night. Sleep is not my friend. The depression continues to crush me. I don't think my body even knows how to make happy endorphins anymore.

I spend so much time in my head now, thinking, spiraling, picking apart the pieces of my life. God is always there, somewhere in the mix of my thoughts, hovering like a question I can't answer. *Why am I on this path? What am I supposed to do with all this pain, all this loss? How do I move forward?*

It took me nearly a year to fill the pages of my first journal. Now I am just a couple of months into this new one, and it feels different but the same—raw, vulnerable, and cathartic, a little like standing in front of a mirror naked, forcing myself to look at the scars. I continue to write, because in some strange way, it's the only thing that reminds me I'm still moving. I document my small victories, my failures, and the random bits of inspiration I find in the chaos, clinging to whatever pushes me forward.

> Journal Entry. I'm questioning everything—God, my faith. Why am I walking through this trial? Two years feels like an eternity, and right now, I can't shake the feeling that my life is slipping through my fingers, wasted. But somehow, I'm still clinging to faith, even if it's just by the thinnest thread.

It's funny—maybe even a little ironic—that it's my faith making me question God. Why me? Why this? Why now? I'm grasping at straws, trying to make sense of what feels like senseless suffering. But in the middle of it all, in the middle of this storm that's threatening to tear me apart, there's this quiet. This strange, steady calm that's still with me, that I can't fully explain.

I shouldn't feel peace right now. Nothing about my life is how I pictured it would be, and yet, here it is—a peace that doesn't match my circumstances. It's a presence that feels too gentle to hold me together, but somehow it does.

Journal entry, July 2012. I can't believe I'm still here—trapped in this broken body, going through medication withdrawal yet again. Even in the middle of all this suffering, I feel a strange sense of peace. And for the first time, I'm starting to picture myself getting better, little by little. "Little by little, a little becomes a LOT."

*   *   *

I'm strong. I'm not broken. I will overcome this. I've written those words onto sticky notes, bright yellow, now folding at the edges, against the dull wall by my bed, as if pinning them there will somehow make them true. Sometimes I even say it out loud, just to see if I believe it more when it hits the air. I ordered an 8x10 print of a powerful, majestic looking horse. A woman by the name of Joni Eareckson Tada painted it with her teeth because she is unable to move her body from the neck down. It rests in a frame on my nightstand, serving as a daily reminder of our vast potential and the importance of never giving up. I've absorbed her words through speeches and interviews, her experience with chronic pain resonating deeply as she speaks of torment and triumph with unwavering faith and a relentlessly positive spirit.

I finished a book today. An entire book. It's strange how something so simple can feel like a victory, but it does. After months of medication withdrawal, months where even holding a thought was a struggle, this feels like proof that the worst is behind me. My mind is quiet enough now to focus, to lose myself in the pages instead of the relentless chaos inside my own body. I sit here, in the corner of my room, surrounded by words and images of strength. Each word pulls me in, reminding me of the connection between mind and body—how they fight, how they heal. And for the first time in a long time, I start to believe in my own ability to rise from this.

SEVENTEEN

HOPE

Healing doesn't follow a neat, predictable path. It loops and stumbles. And just when you think you've run out of energy, time or both, suddenly, everything clicks. And you allow yourself to become cautiously optimistic that, just maybe, you've finally got a handle on the pieces of your life. What was once shattered, seems to be coming together. But then, just as quickly, they explode again, scattering in ways that make no sense, leaving you lost and bewildered, grasping at thin air.

Healing isn't some shiny thing you can grab off a shelf and buy with your privilege, talent, or connections. No, it takes a relentless grit. And it requires you to dig. You dig until your hands bleed and your soul's screaming for you to stop. "Just give up!!!" Every ounce of your being wants to, but somewhere inside you know you have to go deeper and deeper until you hit the bottom, the parts of yourself that you never wanted to see.

I spent so long waiting. Waiting to wake up one morning and just be . . . healed. I thought one day I'd feel like I was supposed to—like any other twenty-something young woman, full of life and energy, bouncing out of bed. I thought I'd get my old body back, the one that didn't constantly remind me of pain and limitations. I had myself convinced that somewhere, out there, there was a magic pill with my name on it that would transform me in an instant, like the fairy godmother did with Cinderella. And the longer my healing stretched on, the more I noticed how people hold tight to the idea of a quick fix, as if there's something out there that can instantly untangle years of pain and all the messes we've made.

I kept searching for that whole and unbroken girl to materialize at first, in every therapy session, in every pill they handed me. But the more I looked, the more I understood—she was gone. The girl who could run and feel invincible, she vanished in the wreck, buried somewhere beneath the shattered glass and twisted metal.

It took time, but I stopped waiting for her to return.

And as strange as it sounds, I don't miss her anymore. Sure, I wish I could feel whole again. I wish the pain would go away and my vitality would return. But that old me, the one who walked through life unaware of how quickly things can change—she's not coming back, and I've come to terms with that.

What I have now is a new understanding of life's fragility, of the gift that health really is. This new perspective—this deep, unshakable gratitude for the simplest things, for breath, for the moments when my pain subsides just a little—those fleeting moments of relief are a gift.

* * *

We arrived in Dallas yesterday and checked into a hotel. My dad is here, and I asked my aunt to come along too. My mom has reached a point where she's just . . . done. The accident, the endless caretaking—it's worn her down in ways I can see even if she doesn't say it. My aunt has stepped in to fill her shoes, and I couldn't be more grateful. We've always shared a close bond, and having her here brings a comforting sense of peace.

I'm sandwiched between my aunt and my dad, perched in a solid ergonomic chair. A giant table stretches out in front of me, polished to a shine, reflecting the faces of people I don't know, in dark suits and crisp ties who look like they are scrutinizing my every move.

There's a blank, white projection screen to my right and a tiny remote on a small table in front of it ready to condense the last few years of my life into pictures—the accident, my pain, my broken body—and neat bullet points to guide the conversation, my pain reduced to topics they can analyze and negotiate over. I struggle to hold my body upright as I shift on my donut cushion, back and forth like a pendulum, as if that tiny movement could somehow ease the ache that's become part of me. I try to focus on the black remote, on anything other than the people in the room and the knot in my stomach that's twisting tighter and tighter. I feel queasy as I think about how I rushed to the hotel bathroom earlier this morning, barely making it before I emptied my stomach into the toilet—a tangled mess of nerves. Today is mediation. I sit here, waiting for my legal team, trying to keep my mind still, but the memories force their way in, fragmenting the past eight months.

I think about what it took to break free of withdrawal, tear myself off that last rung of dependence and walk, while slightly unsteady, free. Eight months since I've been medication-free, and it still doesn't feel real. But the truth is, I'm still in a lot of pain— married, in a way, to ice packs, heating pads, and a compact metal block that sends waves to my nerves in an effort to alleviate pain. I go through bottles of Biofreeze like they're cheap perfume, and the smell of menthol always clings to me.

After I came off the painkillers, I felt the weight of it all settle into my body—the healing I still had to do was vast. I could finally think clearly enough to face it, and I knew I had to dig deeper. In between doctors' visits, physical therapy, and meetings with my lawyers, I researched like my life depended on it. Because it did. I wasn't just scrolling for answers while in the doctor's waiting room to kill time; I was starving for information that would alleviate my pain. Functional medicine was still a mystery, barely gaining any traction and buried under the mainstream's quick-fix solutions. There was no Instagram influencer with a wellness protocol on a silver platter within my reach. I was on my own, scraping up scraps from the corners of the internet, stumbling onto the words "root cause medicine" wondering what the heck that meant. These certainly were not terms I encountered in my formal education in nutrition, and I quickly realized there were many gaps to fill. Hitting the gym and monitoring my protein intake wasn't going to cut it anymore, not after the accident. What used to keep me strong was useless now. This was different; healing would demand something bigger, something drastic.

At first, I clung to one supplement after another, cycling through bottles, convinced that somewhere inside those capsules lay my salvation. It felt almost comforting to believe that a single pill—at least this time a natural one—could restore me, patch up the parts of myself that felt irreparably broken. But it was as if my body knew better than I did. Magnesium, fish oil—it all slipped right through me, weaving its way through the cracks that my shattered body was desperate to heal, leaving the damage untouched; like my body was unable to absorb what I was taking in.

I bought binders, notebooks, highlighters—anything to hold the information I was gathering. I delved into countless dietary theories, collecting books on everything from plant-based ways of life to carnivore diets. My days turned into pages, filled with notes I scribbled from the endless rabbit holes I fell down. Then I discovered Dr. Andrew Weil, a medical doctor who uses a more holistic approach to healing. When I landed on his website, I felt this full-body knowing and I didn't just read his words; I drank them in. The way he talked about restoring homeostasis in the body made something click inside my brain. His motto, "A toxic body is a painful body," became mine: I underlined it, highlighted it, etched it into my memory. It was the answer I didn't know I needed. It took some time for me to realize that he wasn't just talking about physical pain, but the toxicity he was referring to also referenced the kind of pain that hides in the shadows—the kind that seeps out as chronic illness, depression, anxiety, crippling fatigue, and so forth.

And there it was—the "rain barrel effect," a term coined by Dr. Stephen Cabral, but frequently used by many functional practitioners. All the toxins, the residue from medications, the traumas, the stress—they pile up until they finally spill over creating an inflammatory storm in the body. It's layered beneath the surface, building up until the body can't handle it anymore. I started to wonder if the agony I felt was caused by more than just the wreckage from my accident. Maybe it wasn't just the injuries. Maybe it was the cumulative weight of years spent battling chronic pain, sleepless nights, immobility, and trauma from the accident and a toxic relationship—all compounded now by the added strain of the lawsuit. It's all theory, sure, but it felt like pieces were coming together and I could sort of make out the picture, like I was finally tracing the outline of my own story. The accident, the CRPS—it was all part of it, but maybe there was more. This type of healing would mean immersing myself fully in the process, diving deep into a detox protocol to cleanse my body, while also unearthing everything within—old wounds, past experiences, and unresolved emotions. I'd need to peel back each layer, one by one, facing whatever comes up with honesty and courage, clearing out everything that no longer served me to rebuild from the ground up. I realized that I am not destined to remain unwell forever! That I had the power to choose how I breathed, thought, moved, and lived, and that every decision I made influenced my well-being—I could either harm or heal my body. By reducing inflammation and creating a healthier internal environment, I could support my body's natural ability to heal itself.

My body was barely holding itself together; like an old machine with its power lines frayed and sparking, I was about to unravel and go limp. It was as though my mitochondria, the tiny engines inside each cell, were just idling, refusing to do more than the bare minimum. And when I sat back and got quiet with myself, I realized I felt poisoned in a way. I was stumbling through each day, clinging to fragments of sentences that slipped through the fog in my brain like smoke. I couldn't hold on to a thought long enough to string it together. And sleep was no remedy. No matter how long I let myself rest, the weight of exhaustion pressed down, every morning dragging me into the day feeling fatigued, confused, fragmented.

I knew the standard American diet I was consuming wasn't helping, that it might even be contributing. My once-resilient digestive system had been destroyed, likely from a combination of medications and stress. My stomach—so sensitive that even a sip of coffee would make me sick—wouldn't allow me to keep anything down that wasn't gentle, bland, stripped of anything I used to enjoy.

I continued ordering book after book, each one offering its own cure-all, claiming to know the way back to health. The pages piled up, promising miracles through food, promising me healing could be mine if I just followed their plan. At first, it was too much, too many conflicting voices. So, I started stripping them down, taking what felt right, leaving the rest behind. I filled three-ring binders with my notes, trying to make sense of it all, like piecing together a map. Slowly, a plan emerged—a plan that felt like mine. I titled it: "Heal and Rebuild."

It was clear to me my body needed a break from processed foods and a strict elimination diet would be necessary for a time. The thought of cutting out pasta and pizza was brutal; it felt like a betrayal, a sacrifice that cut deeper than any restriction ever had. But I'd do it. I'd do anything to reclaim my health. Because more than pizza, pasta, or chocolate cake—I wanted my life.

I was mindful of every bite I'd take from sunrise to the moment I shut my eyes at night. Whole foods, and only whole foods. Everything I put in my body would serve a purpose: to fuel healing, to start reversing the damage I'd let creep into every cell. Food would be my medicine.

Living with my parents meant my 'pantry' was a closet, and anything that needed to stay cold was stashed in the outdoor fridge. But I preferred it that way. It kept my food in order, and I quickly realized that sticking to a diet like this demanded a level of organization I hadn't needed before.

I tore through the kitchen, purging every packaged, every boxed and bagged bite with ingredients that read like a foreign language. One by one, I pitched every so-called "healthy" option— every package with a little green checkmark or a label that had promised wellness. It hit me, hard: they could slap a "healthy" stamp on anything now. Healthy Cheerios. Healthy granola bars. All-natural frozen Lean Cuisines.

"I'm going to be in the kitchen experimenting a lot!" I told my mom, brimming with a reckless optimism I'd yet to earn.

Mom gave a quiet, almost hidden smile, saying nothing. But I could sense it—a silent hope buried beneath her calm expression, wishing my efforts would pay off, even though she held back from fueling my own hopes.

At first, I fumbled my way through it. The failures came quickly. I remember the first green smoothie I made—the thick, sludge-like texture, the earthy smell that made my stomach turn before I even took a sip. I forced it down, or tried to, the bitter flavor exploding across my taste buds. I gagged, pushing it away. *How was I supposed to do this?* I loved food. I loved the way it brought people together, the way it tasted, the joy it brought—and this . . . this wasn't that. I knew if I was going to be able to sustain this self-imposed journey, I'd have to find a way to make the foods I prepared taste good.

Food was part of my healing journey, sure, but it was just one piece of the puzzle. I started adding new rituals to my day. I thought of them as lifestyle remedies. Small adjustments that, in the moment, felt insignificant—like trying to stop the rain by holding out a single hand. But I hoped, somehow, that these tiny shifts would stack up, that they would yield great results if I just stayed the course.

I kept reading, kept searching for answers, reaching beyond my own culture, trying to find something—anything—that might guide me to a pain-free life of thriving. What I found were other ways of living, unfamiliar paths to healing that were worlds apart from how we did things in America. The Finns especially captivated me with their rituals of detox, rooted in the deep heat of infrared saunas. There was something sacred about it, something I could almost feel, calling to me through the pages. I signed up for a year-long course in alternative medicine, and when infrared saunas came up again, I knew right then that this had to be part of my daily rhythm, a ritual to shed what no longer served me.

My dad and I were eating breakfast together one morning and I couldn't get the sauna off my mind. Before I knew it, the words came spewing out in between sips of my blueberry smoothie. "I need an infrared sauna," I pleaded with him, dramatic as ever, "or I'm going to die!" I punctuated it with short syllables to get the point across.

It wasn't just about the sauna; it was about feeling like my body might give up on me if I didn't start taking drastic measures beyond food. We found a used one on eBay and ordered it.

I continued with the online course and dug into every bit of information I could find as I waited on my sauna to arrive. I wanted to heal so deeply. I wanted to enjoy food again without consequences. I wanted to do something as simple as wake up and get myself ready for the day and have coffee with a friend without my body paying for it dearly.

Before I knew it, my kitchen became somewhat of a lab, as I continued to experiment with whole foods, juicing fresh fruits and vegetables, making nutrient-dense soups and smoothies and my own herbal tinctures and infusions. I would eat big bowls of melons and pineapples in one sitting for the digestive benefits. I even tried making a homemade pizza crust out of almond flour and dairy-free cheese. It was at least edible. I knew my goal was to lower the inflammation in my body so I could add the foods I loved, in moderation, back into my weekly rotation someday.

I decided to go completely gluten-free after reading stories of others who had improved pain with a gluten-free diet. Back then, gluten-free was barely a whisper that could only be heard in hardcore hippie health stores. I remember wandering the aisles, discovering one sad box of noodles that, when I got home, tasted like cardboard. People turned their noses up at me for this "weird" diet, as if it was some vanity-seeking aesthetic-improving routine I was proselytizing. What they didn't understand was that I was so desperate to feel better, I would have eaten dirt daily if it meant freedom from the pain.

I kept going, harder and harder, only thinking about fueling my body and prioritizing on-going cleansing with my dietary choices. My mom laughed one day when she surveyed my newest haul from the health food store laid out on the counter and said, "You've always been the one to go all-in. If they told you an apple a day would help, you'd eat twenty." She was right.

I began a supplement regimen focused on pain relief, detoxi-fication, and supporting mitochondrial health. Instead of begrudg-ingly popping pain pills all day, I found myself proudly downing these horse-sized capsules. It felt empowering to fuel my body in a way that was actually helping it heal.

And then the day I had been waiting for finally arrived—my infrared sauna showed up in an immense box on our doorstep. It's a large one-seater, vertical design, made of cedar, and I could smell the fresh scent of wood as my dad unpacked the box. I started using it that very day, like a kid on Christmas morning, I could hardly wait. I'd been reading about the endless benefits, convinced it would help with the nerve pain, and would bring me to a level of healing I was craving. But nothing prepared me for how sick I was going to feel in those first sessions. The migraine would hit almost immediately, along with waves of nausea and dizziness. My whole body would ache relentlessly, similar to how it feels when you have the flu. I later learned that the heat wasn't just bringing sweat to the surface; it was stirring up toxins hidden in the body, flushing them from my tissues where they'd buried themselves. My system, overwhelmed, fired back with this "healing crisis"—a detox reaction, the body's own wild protest at being forced to let go. My body was so fragile and depleted that I could only tolerate sitting in it for ten minutes at a time. But still, I kept coming back to it, sometimes twice a day, finally working my way up to forty minutes.

There were also IVs, cocktails of vitamins, minerals, and glutathione dripped into my veins week after week. I tried Eastern, Western, Ayurvedic, traditional Chinese medicine—pulling bits and pieces from each, grasping onto anything that might hold an answer. I was desperate, gathering hope from whatever source seemed to offer it. I started intensive chiropractic and alternative pain management sessions with a doctor who had a new approach to pain and together we came up with a game plan that seemed promising. My goal was to never put another pain pill in my mouth again—even if it meant doing this type of therapy for the rest of my existence.

Four times a week for over a year I showed up, grinding through physical therapy and pain management. My mom and sister had taken turns shuttling me to all my appointments because my right leg was still compromised by the paralysis. They'd helped me so much, but I knew if I ever wanted my independence back, I'd have to face the fear that had settled over me like a second skin. I had to drive again—not just around the block in a mock-attempt but everywhere and with intention.

I reached for the keys hanging by the garage door, gripping my donut cushion in the other hand. "I'm driving myself to therapy today," I announced casually to my mom, who was just finishing her coffee.

She froze, and I saw it—the fear in her eyes, a helplessness she couldn't mask. I steadied myself. "I'm going," I said softly. "I can do this." She looked at me as if she wanted to argue, to tell me to wait, to stay, but the words didn't come. She knew it was useless. I'd made up my mind. And maybe she understood, in that deep place only a mother knows, that this was how it had to be. She had to let go of me as if I were a small child all over again.

I forced myself onto the main roads, alone, wrestling with anxiety each time I turned the key. Because of the paralysis in my right leg, I had to teach myself to drive with my left, my foot awkwardly stretching for the gas and brake, compensating for the dead weight of my paralyzed right leg. It felt strange at first, but

I managed. Slowly, almost without realizing it, that drive became my own kind of freedom. I remember the first time I stopped at a coffee shop on the way back from physical therapy, stepping out of the building with a warm cup in my hand, opening up the driver's side door and climbing in behind the wheel. I smiled, basking in the gentle shock of normalcy as it settled over me. It felt so simple. So ordinary. So unbelievably good.

I ran into an old friend about four months into that eight-month journey of detox and trying to bring myself back to life. She hadn't seen me in almost a year. I'll never forget how she looked at me, "It's like there's life in you again," she said, as if I were a ghost that had somehow found its way back to flesh and blood.

"Whatever you're doing," she told me, "keep it up."

Her words cracked something open in me. I held it together in front of her, but as soon as I was alone in my car, I let the tears come. I cried because I knew—I knew that something was working, that all those hard, endless days were adding up to something real. One morning, I woke up and immediately sensed it. No crushing fatigue. No flu-like haze dragging me down. The pain was still there but I was having longer moments of relief. I whispered a quiet thank you to God, and the tears came again—this time, happy ones. It was like I'd found the door back into my own life. And I wasn't beating my head against it anymore. I was walking through it on my own strength, independently.

I started to feel a spark again—like life was slowly finding its way back into my broken body. All I could think was, *If this is working for me, then what could it do for someone else?* I knew I wanted to help people, to share whatever this strange, hard-won alchemy was. I started sketching out a plan, piecing together a path I hadn't even known I wanted. Before the accident, my focus was on fitness and exercise science, but since then, my passion had shifted toward leveraging nutrition and lifestyle to heal the body. I wanted to go back to school, get a master's degree, and continue to learn everything I could about how to heal people from pain.

But even as this vision of the future took shape, there was still a shadow lurking behind me. The lawsuit. It was everywhere, bleeding into every corner of my life, filling me with anxiety. I'd become paranoid, convinced "they"—the other side—were watching me. My lawyers had warned me it was a possibility, and after that, I noticed unfamiliar cars parked across the street from our house, just enough times to make me feel uneasy. Most days, I'd hang a beach towel over the glass in the front door, a flimsy shield against the feeling that eyes were on me, waiting to catch me in some act they could twist to benefit their case against me.

Chronic pain is invisible, I'd remind myself, *but that doesn't stop it from consuming you.* If they snapped just one photo of me hobbling down the street, that single image could be damning. But that would just be a snapshot. They'd never see the full picture of what my life had been reduced to over the past three years.

I started seeing a counselor during that time to help me through the difficulty of navigating a lawsuit, as well as to process all the trauma I had endured. I'd thought I'd already covered all the stages of grief, that I'd dug through the rubble of everything I'd lost, but she showed me I had one step left: acceptance. I'd come to it on my own, somewhere along the way, but she helped me really face it. We peeled back layers of trauma I hadn't realized I was still carrying, the kind that sits heavy in your bones and muscles, deep down in places you forget to look. I did a lot of crying and processing on my part. Every session, I felt a little lighter, a little stronger, like I was letting go of things I'd held on to for far too long.

As I continued the relentless march of physical therapy, I chronicled each victory. From barely able to use a stationary bike to the fluid strides on an elliptical, and finally, the pinnacle of rehabilitation: being able to walk for fifteen minutes on a treadmill, unassisted. Learning to trust my body again was a mental challenge in itself. I remember the first walk I took by myself from the house to the neighborhood cul-de-sac and back. I grabbed my small dog and held onto his leash like a security blanket. I had never felt more grateful for the simple freedom to move.

Over time I noticed changes in my right leg and foot—it was subtle, yet miraculous, watching as the movement and sensation slowly crept back in. I could finally wiggle all my toes in my right foot again. You don't realize how much you rely just on your toes to get you around, until you don't have use of them. I made a bold choice. Against my doctor's counsel, I abandoned the orthotic that had clung to my leg far too long for my liking. The orthotic was not only incredibly uncomfortable, it was a daily reminder of my disability. I wanted it gone. I thought getting rid of it would force me to learn to use that leg again—would somehow wake up the nerves that were damaged. I also understood the risk. I knew I'd be leaving that ankle exposed, fragile, one wrong move from breaking.

The first time I ventured brace-free out to the mall with a friend I was clad only in flip-flops. I'll never forget watching my right flip-flop soar through the air in an act of rebellious liberation and skid across the floor, leaving me barefoot and doubled over in laughter. I quickly understood the need for tennis shoes; not just to keep my shoe on my foot, but to avoid an unceremonious face-plant.

I tried many alternative therapies on my healing journey. Cryotherapy. Colon hydrotherapy. Acupuncture. Neuromuscular massage. I even started sessions in hyperbaric oxygen chambers to help with pain and promote whole-body healing. Anything that might numb the pain and restore my health, I tried it. I read about methylated B vitamin injections used as an alternative solution for chronic pain patients—apparently designed to target nerve pain right at the root. Without a second thought, I jumped on my computer, combing through websites, calling clinics, searching for anyone who could give me the shot. Each call was another disappointment; most doctors didn't even know what I was talking about, let alone offer a willingness to try it. Finally, I found one doctor an hour away from my hometown. I called her, and by the next week, I was standing in her office, holding a vial of the solution I'd take home with me and inject myself with. I was so nervous about giving myself the shot that I decided to numb my hip with ice first. Surprisingly, the ice helped. I'll never forget that first injection—the way it washed over my inflamed body with a cooling sensation. I couldn't believe it. I just laid in my bed, my body completely and totally relaxed. It worked.

I wanted to shout it from the rooftops—these lifestyle mod-ifications and treating food as medicine was truly healing me. But instead, I became selective—almost guarded about who I talked to about this path I was on. It didn't take long to see that my journey, this winding, alternative road, was strange to most people. Many didn't want to hear it, and so shut me down at the first sign of our conversation approaching a topic that veered off the beaten path of conventional medicine. I got it; I believed in modern medicine too. It saved my life. But why couldn't there be room for both? I wanted everyone to see what I was seeing, the small transformations, the hope that replaced the most basic existence of survival. It also hit me along the way that most people don't know what it truly takes to heal a broken body. Real healing isn't a single pill or a quick fix; it's slow, relentless work. It's individual, tailored to each scar, each line of pain. It takes time—sometimes, oftentimes, years.

After months on a waiting list, I finally got an appoint-ment with a naturopathic doctor. When I left their office after the appointment, I half expected to be a pint low on blood with all the vials they took. I was learning that functional medicine was thorough, leaving no stone left unturned. These doctors are detectives, peeling back the layers of symptoms, driven to find the root cause of my pain. They weren't just looking for inflammation; they wanted to know why I was inflamed. Real holistic care looks at everything—the stress, the sleep, the trauma etched into your body. The tests weren't just routine; the ranges they used were narrower, more exacting.

The results came in—blood, urine, stool, saliva, ultrasound. I found out my thyroid had been "shredded" in the accident, just torn apart by the whiplash. For years, I'd been living with barely any thyroid function, which made sense. I was also on the verge of adrenal failure, meaning my hormones were a chaotic mess. My body had been slowly shutting down, piece by piece. Leaving my liver barely hanging on.

The diet and lifestyle changes I'd made were helping, keeping me going, but the years following the accident had done a lot of damage to my body, and it was clear I needed more time. I understood the importance of proper testing to truly pinpoint deficiencies and areas of weakness in my body, and only wished I would have done it sooner. When I walked out of that office, my doctor looked me in the eye and said, "You're going to keep getting better and better." I couldn't remember the last time anyone had said that to me. Most would glance at my medical history, see the X-rays, and treat me like a lost cause. But not her. This doctor validated me, she believed in me, and most importantly, in the possibility of healing. And that gave me one of the greatest healing tools of all: *hope.*

*   *   *

The door swings open, and there he is—the man I'd only met once, the day he flew from Texas and showed up at my door for our first meeting. He was the Texan lawyer my local law team had hand picked to argue my case since all court proceedings would occur in Texas. That day, he'd greeted me with a bear hug that had caught me off guard, and I liked him right away. Since then, we'd spoken just a handful of times over the phone and on Zoom, and honestly, I never thought he'd take my case. But here he is, this giant of a man, the type who went to war for those who'd been taken advantage of, who fought on behalf of survivors. I'd heard he'd been awarded by Oprah and celebrated by Ellen for his courage in taking on high-profile child abuse cases. Some referred to him as a "bulldog in the courtroom," the kind of person you didn't want to go up against.

As he walks in, my body relaxes. He is a big guy in a navy suit and a light blue tie, his eyes kind. He gently pats me on the shoulder, then sits beside me, and I notice the quiet in the room, the way everything seems to still when he enters. It feels surreal, like I am watching a scene from someone else's life, not mine. I glance down at the table in front of him. He has nothing—no notes, no folders. My mind spins, thinking he'd have a mountain of papers, all organized and ready.

I lean over, whispering, "Do you have notes?"

He smiles, a knowing grin, and winks. "I don't need notes."

I flush, feeling the smallest smile tugging at my lips.

Across the table sits Dave's father. Earlier, he greeted me with a kiss on the head—a gesture that, I later learned, had pissed off one of my lawyers. Dave was down the hall in a separate room, as I'd requested to avoid contact with him. One by one, people around the table begin to speak, each taking their turn. Finally, my lawyer speaks. His presentation is captivating, powerful. It is also incredibly hard for me to sit through. My health has improved, sure, but the stress of the lawsuit is taking its toll. Pain is always there, always a reminder. Just sitting in the room is a struggle. I don't take pain medications anymore—just a TENS unit clipped to my side and ice packs in a cooler down the hall. All I can think about is sinking into a bed and reclining.

The presentation opens with videos of me in the life I used to know—snow skiing, deep-sea fishing with my dad, running, dancing. There's even a clip of me doing backflips at the University of West Florida gym, dressed in athletic gear. My lawyer points out my muscular physique, then turns to the opposing lawyer and asks if he has ever had abs like that.

Each image hits me like a punch to the gut, and I fight back tears. Then come testimonials from surgeons, one predicting my future and estimating my life expectancy. It isn't hopeful. One of my surgeons crushes a Styrofoam cup, just like he did for me once, to illustrate the trauma my body has endured. My lawyer speaks about the severity of my injuries, painting a picture of a future I can't bear to imagine. I want to scream, "No, that's not going to be me!"

He reaches into his briefcase and pulls out a small, blue handheld roller, holding it up for everyone to see. "This here," he says, "this device is part of her daily routine now. She uses it, along with the smooth edge of butter knives, anything she can find to break up the scar tissue that covers her body. The first time I had the pleasure of meeting Caitlin I immediately took note of the bruises on her neck and shoulders. She bruises herself, rubbing so hard she's black and blue, desperate to drive the pain away." He pauses, glancing at the group. "This young woman . . . is always wearing a TENS unit or wrapped in ice packs that have left burn marks on her body; she is in and out of hot baths all day, just to manage the pain and keep her head above water without pain medication. Would you choose this life?" he asks, his voice cutting through the silence as he faces the opposition.

Not a single response.

He continues. "She spends hours at therapy each week to help her maintain some sort of quality of life." His voice softens. "And trust me, you don't want to hear about the road she went down with those drugs—the horrific withdrawal she fought through. I don't think anyone in this room can imagine what that took."

The final piece of his presentation is a video from a mock-jury session held the previous week. The jurors knew the details of my case, every brutal bit of it. My lawyer played them the police recording from the night of the accident. I had no idea a tape even existed. I am not prepared for it. In the video, you can hear me, barely conscious, slipping in and out, screaming blood curdling screams caused by the indescribable pain. And then, there is silence before the screams start up again. In the background, Dave is talking to the police, laughing as he casually recounts the events. The sound of his laugh makes me want to vomit right there in front of everyone. I see the jurors on the screen, tears in their eyes, some of them appear visibly angry.

I lose it. I lay my head down on the table and sob, my body shaking uncontrollably. I'm having a panic attack. My aunt and dad help me out of the room, leading me down the hall to a quieter space where I can breathe through it. I just cry and cry, letting it all out.

My lawyer wraps up his statement, and my hometown lawyers, who'd come along to support me, whisper that it was brilliant. Negotiations go back and forth, both sides holding firm. We stay in a hotel nearby, waiting, the tension almost unbearable.

Two days later, the phone rings. My dad recognizes the area code, motioning for me to come over. He puts it on speaker, and we listen together.

"We won," is all I hear my lawyer say.

I collapse onto the couch, covering my face with my hands, whispering, "Thank you, God!" over and over again. I glance up to see my dad's face, and for the first time in my life, I see him cry. I sob, "I can't believe it, I can't believe it!" Waves of relief mix with disbelief, like all the pain and stress is seeping out, leaving me hollow and free.

In the weeks following the close of my case, I swing between an emotional high and a deep physical and mental exhaustion. I sleep a lot, and sometimes, out of nowhere, I start to cry, as if years of pent-up burdens are finally breaking free. There's a profound sense of gratitude, but a part of me feels undeserving. What about all the other patients I met along the way? Will they find relief, be cared for, and receive compensation for their suffering? It's a question I know I'll always carry with me.

My dad's friend had called my lawyers the "dream team," and I guess he was right. For the first time, I feel truly validated. My injuries, my pain—it was and is real. Catastrophic. Despite what others were trying to make me believe. I find myself repeating it, like a mantra, almost like I still don't believe it: We won.

EIGHTEEN

16,404 FEET

I stand in my childhood bedroom, the floor scattered with clothes, sentimental trinkets, and boxes that I have half-heartedly packed. Today is the day. After years of being confined in this room . . . this house—by my pain, trauma, and the weight of my own broken body—I am finally stepping into a life of my own making. A new home. My own space. I should be excited. And I am mostly. But beneath it all lies a quiet undercurrent of anxiety, subtle yet persistent.

What if I am not ready? What if I can't do this? What if the pain is too debilitating for me to be on my own? My mom hovers in the doorway, arms crossed, her face painted with concern.

"Are you sure you're ready for this?" she asks for the hundredth time. "How are you going to take care of everything? Yard work, cleaning . . . living?" Her voice is gentle but edged with worry, the kind only a mother can master.

I pause, a shirt clutched in my hands, and turn to her. "I don't care if I have to Ace bandage ice packs to my back all day long." I try to make it sound like a joke, and it comes out sounding much more resolute than I feel. "I have to do this. It's now or never." My voice cracks just enough for her to catch it, but I don't let her linger on it. "Besides," I add with a smile, "Nick will be there. He can handle the heavy lifting." My cousin, who is also a close friend and someone I share so many childhood memories with, will be staying in the guest bedroom while completing his master's degree. I won't be alone.

Mom smiles despite herself, but her eyes shine with tears she won't let fall. I know what she isn't saying. She has been not only my mother but my primary caretaker for three years. From helping me get dressed, to preparing meals to eat when I couldn't manage, as well as guiding me through the pain, trauma, and recovery following my accident—she and I have been through so much together. Letting go is hard for her. I understand, maybe more than she realizes, because letting go is hard for me too. "What are you doing with those clothes?" she asks, gesturing to the pile on the floor. "Trash," I say flatly. "All of it."

Her brow furrows, her eyes assessing the mountain of fabric. Stacks of baggy black pants I had worn to physical therapy. Shirts that reminded me of doctor's appointments. The uniform of a life I wanted so badly to leave behind. "I can't stand to look at them," I explain. "They're part of . . . all of it."

She nods slowly. "Yeah, I get that."

It feels like a necessary purge. Healing, even. Every scrap of that old life needs to go. I'd even bought new sheets—colorful ones, because the white ones I had been sleeping on reminded me too much of a hospital bed.

I tape up another box, sealing its edges with a sharp snap. As I turn to grab the last roll of packing tape, my eyes land on the frame perched on my nightstand that's offered comfort since my hard months of detox. The majestic horse stands frozen midstride, framed by the words: "He gives strength to the weary." I let out a sigh and reach for it. Pressing the frame against my chest, I close my eyes and let the lump in my throat rise and fall. This is what thankfulness feels like—bigger than words, deeper than breath. And I'm overcome by it.

I tuck the frame gently into the last box, surrounding it with soft clothes, and tape the lid shut. My hands linger on the edges of the box as if it held more than just belongings. It feels like it holds everything—the pain, the healing, and the gentle promise of a life I can finally start living.

My parents finish loading the last of the boxes into the back of Dad's truck. I stay in the doorway, staring into the room that once felt like a cage; physically by the hospital bed and mentally by the pain medications. This space had held me like a body cast, locking me in place while I fought to find a way back to myself. But just like a cast is meant to keep a broken bone still in order for it to heal even stronger in the aftermath, I know, too, that my heart has healed, the cracks lined with a resilience that will always be my baseline.

The walls are bare now. The bright, yellow sticky notes are gone—the scriptures, the affirmations, the words I scribbled down in my most desperate moments, to remind myself I was still here, still fighting, are now etched in my mind, and I don't need them anymore because they are as close to me as my own breath. I used to read them over and over, desperate for them to mean something, to save me from the pain and turmoil I was once in. My eyes trace the corners of the room, and it all comes back at once. The nights spent staring at the ceiling, the pain so constant it became its own kind of silence. The tears that burned hot and furious until they didn't come at all. The breaking, over and over, until breaking became the only thing I knew how to do.

This room saw all of it. The darkest days, when even hope felt out of reach, and the quiet victories that kept me going when I was almost out of strength. These walls were the witness to the first time I managed to sit up on my own and the endless minutes I stood gripping my walker, fighting through blinding pain, knuckles white, and the day I took that first, shaky step all on my own. Every moment, no matter how small, mattered here.

I fell apart here, but I also rebuilt myself here. Slowly. Painfully. Piece by piece.

I take one last look around the room, wanting to sear every detail into my memory. Not because I want to dwell on what happened, but because I never want to forget how far I've come.

Settling into the new place doesn't take long. My dog and the stray cat I somehow inherited are already making themselves at home. My cousin is moved in too, and the sound of our laughter fills the house. It reminds me of our childhood and it feels so good to laugh again, to feel lightness after years of carrying so much heavy weight on my shoulders.

But it's not all sunshine and fresh starts. My mom's words echo in my mind, her worry woven into every syllable: *How are you going to manage?* She's not wrong. Chronic pain turns the simplest tasks into mountains. The other day, my dog threw up all over my bed and I tried to change the sheets. Just pulling the fitted sheet over the mattress left me gasping, my body screaming in pain. I couldn't do it. I had to ask my cousin for help. For a moment, the familiar tide of defeat started to rise, the thoughts of failure creeping in. *Pathetic*, they whispered. *You haven't made any progress at all.* But this time, I shoved them back. *No. Not today. I can't put the sheets on my bed now, but one day, I will.* Every night, I cook dinner for myself with an ice pack strapped to my back, held in place by an Ace bandage. By the end of the day, it feels like I can barely keep myself upright—like my body just might break in half.

In the early mornings, before the world is up, I sit on the back porch with a cup of green tea warming my hands, watching the sky come alive in streaks of gold and pink. The air is still, and for a moment, so am I. This is the time I've carved out for myself, a quiet pause to reflect on all I am grateful for. Gratitude has become a powerful perspective shifter for me, changing the way I see and navigate the world. There are still days when the pain crashes over me, so intense that staying in bed feels like the only option to choose—but somehow, I still find the strength to get up. I've learned that even on the hardest days, there's always something to be grateful for. It's not about denying the pain or pretending it isn't real. It's about shifting my focus.

As I sip my tea, I think about how I've been told, more times than I can count, what I wouldn't be able to do after my accident. And yet, here I am, doing those very things. Walking unassisted. Living a life free of painkillers. Healing my body through alternative methods. At some point, I realized that when I let others' perceptions shape how I saw myself, their limitations had the potential to become my reality. The more I observed this process, the more I realized I gave my power away. I refuse to let that happen anymore. I understood the doctors' source for their predictions—they were rooted in data. But I wasn't interested in becoming a statistic. I was determined to prove everyone wrong—not by ignoring the challenges, but by choosing not to let them define me.

One of the most challenging aspects of this healing journey has been my mind clinging to the memory of the athletic woman I once was—craving the days of lifting heavy weights and running with ease while my body refuses to cooperate, even still. It's a humbling experience, to say the least. I've pushed myself in ways I never imagined, but I've also had to unlearn the deeply ingrained mindset that no pain really and truly means no gain, because letting go of my ego isn't a sign of weakness. It doesn't matter what other people think. If I keep forcing my body—trying to do things it is not ready for by trying to rush the timeline—I'll only drag out the healing process farther. There has to be a balance. I have to slow down, to be intentional, in order to hurry the healing process along. As is with all of life—the harder I pushed, the weaker I grew. The more I listened and let go, the stronger I became. For someone who was used to finding my joy in pushing the limits, in feeling the ache of hard work in my muscles, that's easier said than done. But I had to shift my focus—maybe I couldn't pump iron anymore, but I could move my legs, thank God. So, I bought a watch to start tracking my steps and decided to begin by walking around my new neighborhood. Five times a day, for ten minutes at a time wasn't much, but it was a start. I even set a timer to remind me to get my daily steps in.

As I finish sipping my tea, I remember this article I recently read about yoga being a form of pain management. I used to swear I'd never do it—too slow, too quiet, too . . . not me. But I found myself about to leave my house to experience my first yoga class based on that article. I arrived a few minutes early to assess the situation. It occurred to me as I gripped my newly purchased purple yoga mat, that I was standing at the entrance of a fitness studio for the first time in over three years. Nerves were tangling my stomach into knots. It felt monumental, like crossing a bridge into a place that used to be as familiar as home, but now felt like uncharted territory. I left my insecurities outside, reminding myself why I was there in the first place: I had come to find another tool I could use to manage my pain. I wanted to move my body so I could heal.

The yoga teacher, who was also a physical therapist, spoke about pain and illness and how we cannot heal when our nervous system is in overdrive. It never occurred to me until then that my body was most likely stuck in a state of fight or flight. Over the next several months, I worked one-on-one with the instructor, learning to breathe in ways that soothed my insides, finding poses that helped me feel safe in my own skin again. Slowly, I learned to trust my body. I started noticing when my body felt tense, or when my heart rate elevated—I even noticed when my shoulders curled inward to protect me. Slowly, I started to let go.

And then, something extraordinary happened. The pain began to ease—not all at once, but in small, quiet ways. My health continued to improve over time; it was subtle, but I documented them every time I felt something new.

My strength is slowly returning. I am elated every time I catch glimpses of muscle definition on my arms and legs in the mirror. My right leg in particular, once stripped of all muscle mass due to paralysis, now reveals the faint outline of a small calf muscle, which I never thought I would see again. I remember the nickname I was given in high school—"Legs;" when my friends in the weight room would compare their calf muscles to mine, and I always came out on top. I laugh to myself as I think back on that memory.

For so long, I'd been stuck in a cycle of chronic stress and immobility, my body compressed and inflamed from too much stillness. Now, with every careful stretch and breath, it is like my body is opening up again, allowing oxygen to flow to places that had been starved of circulation for years. I now realize how much my nervous system has been holding me hostage, how much my pain was tied to the state of my mind and body working against each other. There have been countless "a-ha" moments along this journey, but this is a big one. Movement isn't just about healing my body, it's about taking my body back. Bit by bit, I feel pieces of myself returning. I smile as I watch myself lift a ten-pound weight in the mirror; I'm coming back to life.

Just as food and movement serve as medicine, so does the act of processing my trauma. I continue to see a counselor as I grapple with the reality that trauma isn't something that can be fixed overnight. It lingers, stubborn and complex, resisting the quick solutions I desperately want to believe in.

I had become an expert in not feeling—because I had to—in order to survive the pain. I had to prioritize my physical feelings and there was just no room for the emotions of surviving. So I packed them all into some deep, unreachable corner and threw away the key. Therapy, I realized, wasn't just important—it was essential. It became a vital piece of my healing puzzle, and what's ironic is that I hadn't even noticed I was missing it. Like finally adding the right ingredient to a recipe I'd been getting wrong for years.

In therapy, we got really focussed on how to reintegrate myself into the real world. After more than three years confined to my parents' house, the idea of stepping back into society felt daunting. Even venturing out alone brought on panic on some days, which was something I couldn't quite shake. Yet, the part of me that yearned to truly live again continued to speak louder than the fear. I'd spent so many years consumed by my pain, but as I sat with my counselor, it hit me—I needed to shift my focus outward, to something bigger than myself if I was going to really and truly heal, all the way.

That week, I picked up the phone and scheduled an interview with a local charity, Big Brothers Big Sisters of Northwest Florida. I hadn't been involved with the organization since high school, but those memories had stayed with me. The power of showing up in a child's life was permanently imprinted on my heart. I quickly threw myself into everything—working galas, helping with charity events, and eventually being interviewed by the local news and sharing my why. I chose to be a part of this organization to further my healing experience and as I was sharing my story with the news crew, it dawned on me: When you serve others, you break free from your own self-pity.

During this time, I decided to finally apply to a master's program in human nutrition. I sent in the recommendations, a written essay, dug up my college transcripts, and waited. A month later, my acceptance letter arrived. Classes started in the fall, just as I'd be finishing my certification in alternative medicine. It felt like the world was finally cracking open again, letting in light.

*   *   *

Another year has passed, a year of digging deep, of peeling back layers and doing the kind of inner work I used to avoid. Healing has woven itself through every part of me—leaving me stronger and more whole than even before the accident.

I sit outside, a warm cup of coffee cradled in my hands as it occurs to me that it's the little moments that carry the greatest meaning. I've missed this—the smell, the taste, the quiet thrill of that first sip. Coffee runs deep in my family; I come from a long line of coffee drinkers, and some of my favorite memories are wrapped in the aroma of freshly brewed cups shared with my grandparents. It was a ritual, a bond, a moment of connection. So when I had to give it up, it felt like losing a piece of myself. For so long, it wasn't even an option. Just the thought of coffee dragged me back to all those moments my stomach turned against me, worn thin by years of stress and painkillers. But today is different. Today, I drink without consequence, without the acid tearing at my insides. I can sit here again, participating in a tradition I thought I'd lost forever.

The morning stretches out in front of me, quiet and unhurried. I'm chatting away with my cousin as we sip our coffees together. The stillness. The conversation. Before the accident, I would've missed it all, too busy rushing to the next thing to see the beauty in what is already here.

I finish my coffee, pull on some athletic gear, and lace up my tennis shoes. It strikes me, as it sometimes does, how normal this feels. Today, I'm participating in a 5K with one of my dearest friends. She's an avid runner, but she's decided to walk with me, matching her stride to mine. It's a kindness I don't have words for.

At the starting line, we stand side by side in matching lime-green shirts. Around us, runners stretch and bounce on their toes, eyeing each other like they're about to compete in the Olympics. The old me would've been one of them, sizing up my competition and turning this into something to conquer. But today isn't about competition. It's about proving something to myself.

We start walking. My friend doesn't rush me, and I don't rush myself. As we move forward, I can't help but reflect on how difficult the journey to this moment has been. I used to define myself as someone who is physical. I was the one who lifted weights, who had the speed of a sprinter, got up when I wanted, and went wherever I pleased. That freedom in that identity was stripped away when I went flying through that windshield at 90 miles per hour. I went from a hospital bed to a wheelchair, then to a walker to regain some sense of mobility. And in the process, I felt like I was becoming a person I didn't want to be—someone who viewed themselves as weak, someone who had become afraid of movement, someone who no longer trusted their own body.

I had to confront those feelings head-on and have a major change in perspective. This shift was likely due to reaching an emotional breaking point, which forced me to reassess what strength looked like. I started to see the walker, not as a symbol of defeat, but as progress—because there had been a time, and not all that long ago, when I couldn't even get out of bed without a crane lifting me into a wheelchair. I forced myself to believe that moving forward, even in the smallest way, was still moving forward. For most people, a 5K might not seem like much. But for me, this is huge. This is proof that I've made progress.

As we reach mile marker 1, I squeeze Jen's hand and say, "I'm ready to run!" She looks at me confused, but replies, "Okay—are you sure?"

"Yes," I respond, "I'm sure!"

We start jogging together. It feels awkward, and I am well aware my form looks ridiculous. A few minutes go by, and I'm still moving. I can't believe it—I'm actually doing it. But then, out of nowhere, I stop. I feel that familiar drag in my right leg. Once paralyzed, it still falters when I've been on my feet too long. The nerves quit firing, and the muscles just refuse to cooperate. It's heavy, unresponsive—I can't move it, not even my toes. It's like trying to move a limb that no longer belongs to me.

I hear my surgeon's words—"You'll never be able to walk more than half the length of a football field without assistance"—ringing in my ears as I limp out of the other runners' way. One hundred fifty feet—that was supposed to be my limit. But today, I walk 16,404 feet. Stubborn as always, I just keep putting one foot in front of the other. And somehow, I make it. I cross the finish line, leg dragging behind me, no brace, no crutch. I nearly collapse at the finish line, but before I do, my friend catches me, steadying me with that big, genuine smile of hers. She wraps me in a warm hug, and we laugh. We did it. We celebrate the only way that feels right—with a meal at our favorite Irish pub.

That night, I lie in bed, restless as the fire in my legs refuses to fade. The ache is sharp, unforgiving, but tonight, it's different. It's earned. I ease my way to the freezer, the cold weight of the ice pack pressed against my body—a victory that's all my own.

NINETEEN

PIECE BY PIECE

The year I start my master's degree is the same year I take on a job doing one-on-one nutrition counseling. It feels right to pour myself into others—people who are hurting, people searching for hope. For the first time in years, my days feel full, overflowing with coaching sessions and even catering health retreats. I'm the busiest I've been since before the accident, and I welcome the pace. Busy feels good. Busy means I'm living, even though the pain lingers. I come to accept that the pain might always be here. But it doesn't consume me anymore; it doesn't dictate the terms of my life. I'm thriving—healthy in a way that matters. I've found purpose, and I have the tools to manage the moments when the pain tries to overtake me.

Not long after, I trade my athletic wear for a formal suit. I'm standing in front of a room full of young professionals, sharing my story at my first corporate wellness event. It feels surreal. I expected to be nervous, but instead, I feel calm, even certain. This is where I'm supposed to be: Where the hurt finds meaning. The words flow easily, and when I finish, the room feels changed. People I don't know line up to shake my hand, to hug me, to tell me their own stories of pain. One woman comes up to me, and with tears streaming down her face, shares her health struggles with me. I hold her hand as she speaks, nodding in understanding, feeling the weight of her words.

When it's over, I walk to my car, climb in, and close the door quickly as I let the sobs erupt from deep within me. I can't believe I'm here, in this moment, after everything. All the pain, all the suffering—it feels as though it's been leading me here. A quiet, profound sense of fulfillment settles over me. It's overwhelming to reflect on where I once was and how far I've come.

The invitations start coming—more events, a few local churches. A local advertising group hears my story and features me in a campaign for the Florida ADDY Awards. To my astonishment, my story takes first place. For the first time, it feels like I'm finally moving in the right direction, and everything is starting to align.

My life revolves around health and wellness now. I spend my days coaching, teaching interactive cooking classes, working a community garden, and catering health retreats for doctors and healthcare professionals at a local hospital. It's demanding, but it's meaningful. Most nights, I come home exhausted, my right leg swollen and solid purple—a telltale sign of complex regional pain syndrome. I drive three hours each month to purchase a vial of solution that I inject myself with to help keep the inflammation at bay. Some days, it feels like a battle I'll never fully win, but I've learned to make peace with it. My health and energy have returned, and that's a gift I'll never take for granted.

Eventually, I step away from catering for wellness retreats. While it is a rewarding experience that allows me to make valuable connections, the long hours on my feet break me down, until I have to surrender. Leaving that chapter behind feels like loosening a too-tight grip. It leaves space, raw and open, for something else. That something arrives in the form of a text: "We're going backpacking in the Montana mountains. Leaving in two days. Want to join?" I don't think, don't pause long enough to second-guess the answer my gut has already decided. *Yes.* Even though I am not sure if I can keep up.

The trip unfolds like a messy, beautiful song. We pile into an old van that smells faintly of gas and adventure, its back stuffed with a cooler and crumpled sleeping bags. We drive aimlessly, stopping wherever the world demands—at the base of jagged peaks, by rivers that shimmer like liquid silver, in wide-open spaces where the sky seems endless. Sometimes we hike, sometimes we picnic, and sometimes we just stand there, in awe of the beauty in front of us. Once, the van breaks down on the side of the road, and we sit in the dust laughing at our bad luck. A kind gentleman helps us get it moving again.

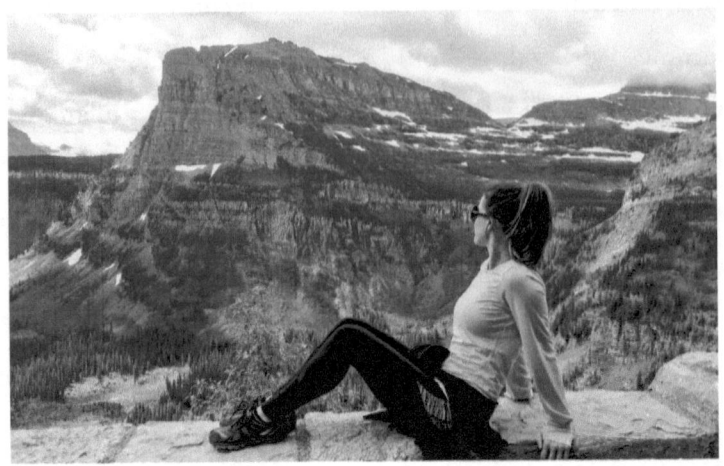

Montana is intoxicating. We venture off-trail more than once, blissfully unaware until a furious park ranger waves us down. "There's a grizzly on the loose," he warns. "It killed someone just two weeks ago." That night, we hole up in a tiny cabin deep in the woods, the walls too thin, our imaginations too loud, picturing something primal lurking just beyond the trees.

After that trip, travel takes root in me like a fever. Over the next year, I find myself planning trips in the spaces between work and school, squeezing adventure into the cracks of my busy life. I roam coast to coast. Each stop unfurls something new to look at, prompting me to feel a corresponding feeling: red rock deserts, stormy gray coastlines, cornfields stretching further than I thought possible. Everywhere I go, I marvel at creation, quietly magnificent, asking for nothing but to be noticed.

When I'm busy navigating a new place, the chronic pain that's always with me feels less overwhelming. Maybe it's the distraction, or maybe it's something deeper—the way being outside in the open air makes my body relax in a way I don't notice until

I'm there. There's something about nature that feels grounding, like it gives me permission to let go of the tension I carry around in my body, without even realizing it. The excitement of the journey releases something in me, a surge of endorphins, and for a little while, the pain fades into the background, my new experiences demanding my attention.

Two years pass, and I find myself living on the beach. Most mornings, I'm on my turquoise bike as the sun rises, pedaling as fast as my legs will take me. The salty breeze whips past my face, and in those moments, I feel untethered to the world, like I'm flying. Sometimes, I tear up on these rides. They're more than exercise—they're therapy, a reminder that I'm here. I'm alive. Today, I ride over twenty miles. It's hard, but I press on. Pain has taught me to respect my limits, but it's also taught me to test them. Every day, rain or shine, I get outside and move my body. I walk along the beach, swim in the mineral-rich ocean—anything to stay connected to the world around me.

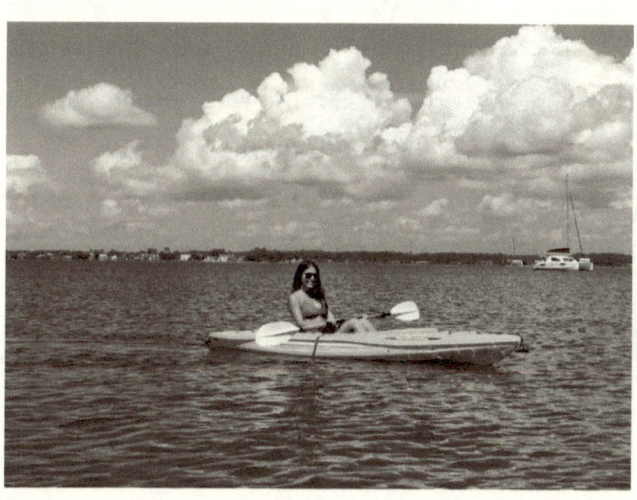

I've started taking dance classes—rumba, East Coast swing, West Coast swing. Last weekend, I slipped into my first pair of low heels in years. They're the kind with straps to keep them from flying off my unreliable right foot. That night, I danced so hard I broke a heel—on my shoe. When I get home that night, I chuckle as I inspect the damage. I decide to keep the shoe; it's a little memento of a night when laughter and movement filled the spaces where pain once overwhelmed my body, mind, and soul.

It feels like I'm finally making up for lost time. I decide to write out a long bucket list in my journal of things I want to do, places I want to see. Koa is on that list; I'd always dreamed of having a golden retriever, like the one that greeted me during my stay at the rehab hospital. The week my golden boy comes into my life, everything shifts.

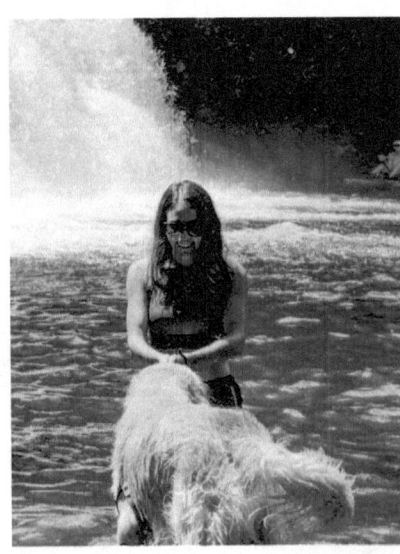

He's always by my side, bounding with energy and a joy that's impossible to ignore. Wherever we go, he comes along too, his bright spirit drawing people in, breaking down walls with just a wag of his tail or the warmth in his eyes. Strangers can't help but smile as he captivates their hearts with his golden energy.

Not long after Koa came into my life, so did another friend. We met when I was in North Carolina, interviewing for an internship. A military guy—kind, genuine, grounded in a way that catches me off guard. When he told me he was a Green Beret, I nodded like I knew what that meant. Later, I googled it. Growing up in a military town around pilots, this was something new to me.

I hadn't dated in a long time, choosing instead to focus on myself. But this guy is different. There's a quiet humility in his voice, a confidence that doesn't need to be shouted to be felt. We connect in a way I didn't think was possible for me. I'd been so broken, I didn't think I'd have the chance to share my life with someone else.

One weekend, he surprises me by flying from North Carolina to Florida just to see me. We sit on the beach, hand in hand in silence, listening to the waves. He turns to me, his eyes steady on mine, and in his best Scottish accent, he quotes, "I love you. I always have."

I laugh. "Braveheart," I reply, smiling at him.

He doesn't know it's my favorite movie, and for a moment, we're caught up in the laughter, swept away by how ridiculous and perfect it all feels. But as the laughter fades, he takes my hand. With a soft, steady voice, he asks me to marry him. There isn't a flicker of hesitation—I say yes. His friends always called him "Superman," and I've always dreamed of marrying Superman.

The very next day, we elope. Just the two of us, a quiet dinner, and a slice of key lime pie on the beach. It's simple. Intimate. Perfect.

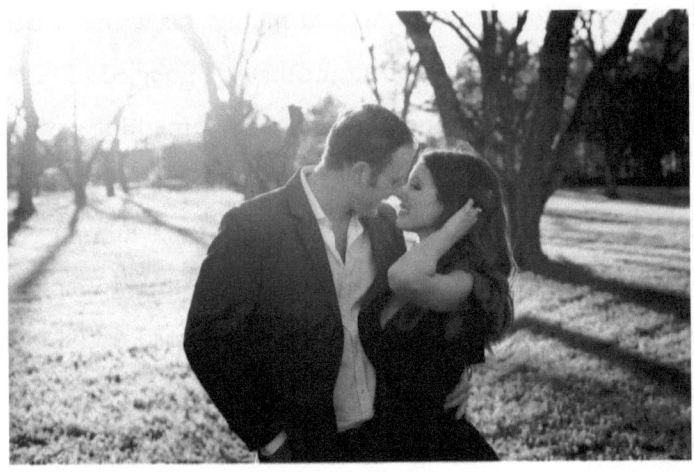

We make plans to move to North Carolina where he's stationed, and I can hardly contain my excitement. North Carolina has always felt like a second home, the place where my family spent countless summers. The mountains, the beaches, the winding trails, the beautiful fall leaves—it holds a piece of my heart that's always been waiting for me to return to. The thought of starting our life together here feels like coming full circle.

Another year passes so quickly—a year filled with joy and discovery. Even now, with tears in my eyes, I still say it was one of the best years of my life. We spend it exploring a new and beautiful place, falling in love with North Carolina and with each other all over again. I'm living a life I never thought I'd get to have. But even in that happiness, there are moments when the weight of everything I've been through catches up to me. I break down like a storm rolling in unexpectedly, and my husband doesn't ask questions. He just pulls me into his arms, holds me tight, and lets me cry. He knows these tears aren't just a result of sadness—they're a reflection of how far I've come and the life we're building together.

Before my surgeries following the accident, the surgeon told my parents I wouldn't be able to have children based on how severely shattered my pelvis was. But as the surgeries proved successful and I recovered better than expected, their certainty softened into a maybe—it would still be difficult, they said. The kind of difficult that made hope feel fragile and dangerous. When we lost our first baby, I didn't know how to talk about it. Sometimes I wonder if it was my body, worn down and malfunctioning from all that it's endured, refusing to do what it was meant to. I take some time to process the miscarriage and everything that comes with it. By spring, I start an internship at a clinic in North Carolina while working to finish my master's degree in human nutrition.

"Come in with an open mind," they tell me on my first day. And I do. I shadow a medical doctor who'd spent over twenty years at the Hippocrates Health Institute in Boston, learning more in those months than I ever thought possible. I hold the hands of patients who are at death's door, watching their lives change as conventional and alternative medicine come together in ways I hadn't seen before. It is eye-opening and humbling. I see life being brought back into bodies that had all but been given up on.

I get to know the patients well. One day, as I help an older woman to the restroom, she turns to me and says, "You look the picture of health." I smile, the compliment landing in a way she can't understand. "Thank you," I respond. "It took me a long time to get here."

She looks at me, confused. "What happened?"

For a moment, I hesitate, but then I share a condensed version of my story. Her eyes fill with tears as she hugs me.

"You give me hope," she says, her voice trembling.

I'll never forget that moment.

I meet so many patients during my time at the clinic. Different faces, all bringing with them unique stories of pain and resilience, all brought to this place searching for the same thing—a better quality of life. These people are desperate for an alternative when everything else has failed.

The year I finish my master's in human nutrition is the same year we welcome our son into the world—our miracle baby. That's what we call him, because for a long time, I didn't think this moment would ever come. As I hold him for the first time, I feel the weight of everything that brought me here. The pain, the endless healing, the fear that sometimes felt bigger than the hope. Every struggle, every step—it all led to this. To him.

*　*　*

Looking back now, it feels surreal to revisit those tough, formative years of my life. They've shaped me in ways I never could have imagined. I know what it's like to hit rock bottom. To lose hope entirely. To stand in the wreckage of your life, feeling like everything you've ever known has been stripped away. Yet somehow—it is possible to find your way back. This kind of journey changes you—it has deeply and permanently altered the way I see the world, myself, and the people around me. Suddenly, the little things aren't so little anymore. You notice them, savor them, hold them close. You don't take anything for granted because you know, in your bones, just how fragile life is, because the pain that came from healing those broken bones still reminds me of this, every day.

*   *   *

In the beginning stages of healing, I did everything by the book. I followed every protocol, every piece of health advice centered around food as medicine, devouring the information and the food with fierce, almost desperate precision. But I learned the stress of trying to adhere to perfection can hinder healing more than it helps. Health needs to be a balance—it should integrate into your life, not overwhelm it.

It also became evident to me as my healing years continued, that mindset acts as its own form of medicine—belief and faith have the ability to spark true healing; coupled with commitment, no matter how desperate, they can be the things that change the whole game, if you let them. I started to believe that my body was strong and capable. My body, intelligently designed, was working for me, not against me. This shift in perspective became pivotal— and was the turning point in my healing journey.

The accident, the trauma, the pain, and the grueling recovery pushed me to redefine who I was physically, mentally, and emotionally. I learned to embrace my vulnerabilities, my scars, but most of all, my pain. At the time, it felt insurmountable, but pain has become my greatest teacher. Suffering taught me resilience. It showed me the strength I didn't know I had. But it also required me to make a critical mindset shift: to stop playing the victim and instead step into the role of a victor. I came to understand that if I stayed stuck in the "why me?" mindset, I would never move forward. Owning my choices and focusing on what I could control became a key component to reclaiming my life.

I discovered that healing isn't a sprint—it's a marathon. There are setbacks and frustrations, moments when you wonder if you'll ever move forward. But you press on. I pressed on. That's what endurance is: showing up for yourself, over and over again, even when it feels impossible. It's okay to rest and take a break, but you just can't quit. Document the small steps—the moments of progress that seem insignificant at first but eventually add up to something profound. I found that embracing the journey instead of obsessing over the end goal is essential. Healing became less about reaching an end point and more about the continuous act of growth. And when I felt defeated, I hit the pause button so I could turn around and look back over all the ground I had covered. Then, I would regain my strength, reminded by just how far I'd come. That perspective gave me the fuel and energy to press on and get me here today.

I realized along the way that no one is going to do it for me. No one is going to hand me all the answers to my healing on a silver platter. Healing is hard work—the hardest work there is. Expect it to be difficult—that's how I formed the mental fortitude to keep going.

My faith has been my anchor through it all. In Christ, I've found a strength that goes beyond my own. I've been bent and broken, but somehow, I've been sustained. God took something that felt irreparable and made it whole again, transforming my pain into purpose. I experienced His love, grace, and compassion in ways I didn't know I needed.

Today, I am filled with a deep sense of thankfulness and awe. I know how fortunate I am to be where I am, and my heart aches for those still suffering in silence, battling their own personal health challenges. My hope is that my story might change the way we think about overcoming trauma, pain, and chronic health struggles—reminding anyone fighting their way through darkness: Don't give up. Hope is a quiet, persistent force, urging us to keep going, even when all we can manage is the next small step forward.

Healing is possible.

*　　*　　*

Eventually, all things find their way, though not as they once were. What was shattered did not mend by time alone. Time watched, but it was faith that lifted me from the devastation and hope that stitched my brokenness into something whole. Not all miracles are instantaneous—some unfold slowly, shaped by quiet grace and an unyielding belief in what could be.

The mountains of Western North Carolina stand before me like sentinels, timeless and unwavering, as I climb the trail. My daughter's small hand rests in mine, warm and sure, a reminder of all I have fought for. Ahead, my husband walks with our son, his laughter drifting through the trees like a song I once feared I would never hear.

I pause to lace up my hiking boot, my body alive with the quiet ache of what it took to get here. The scars I carry no longer feel like burdens, but stories—pieces of a life shattered and rebuilt. The girl I was is gone, but in her place stands a woman of unshakable faith, who has learned that even broken things can be made new again.

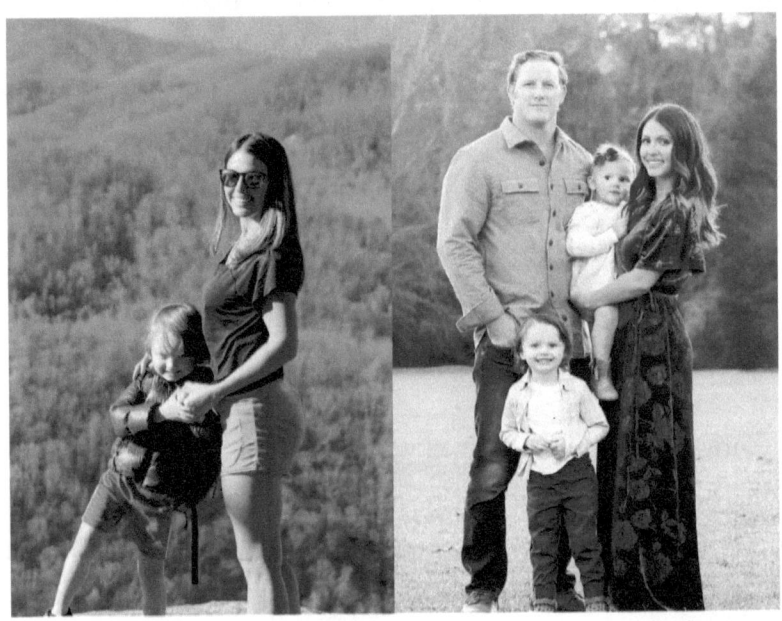